CONTENTS

ISSUES OF INDIAN HEALTH AND HEALTH CARE REFORM

FRIDAY, APRIL 8, 1994

U.S. SENATE,
COMMITTEE ON INDIAN AFFAIRS,
Shiprock, NM

The committee met, pursuant to notice, at 3 p.m. at Shiprock, NM, Hon. John McCain (vice chairman of the committee) presiding.

Present: Senators McCain and Domenici.

STATEMENT OF HON. JOHN McCAIN, U.S. SENATOR FROM ARIZONA, VICE CHAIRMAN, COMMITTEE ON INDIAN AFFAIRS

Senator McCAIN. Thank you very much for your kind words of welcome.

I would like to welcome all of you to this hearing of the Senate Indian Affairs Committee. I would like to point out that I am very pleased not only to be here for myself, but also to be here with Senator Pete Domenici, who is a very dear friend, and frankly, I do not know a better friend of Native Americans in the entire Congress of the United States. I have confidence in Senator Domenici, and it's a great pleasure for me to be with him.

I will make a brief statement, I would like to ask Senator Domenici to make a brief statement, and then we will hear from our first panel of witnesses, which will be composed of the Honorable Jon Kyl, who is a member of Congress from Arizona who represents a large segment of Navajo country in my State of Arizona; Peterson Zah, President of the Navajo Nation; and Genevieve Jackson, Councilwoman and Chairperson of the Health and Social Services Committee of the Navajo Tribal Council; Marshall Plummer, Vice President of the Navajo Nation; and Judy Knight-Frank, who is Chairperson of the Ute Mountain Ute Tribe.

The next panel after that is going to be John Hubbard, who is the Director of the Navajo Area Indian Health Service. And following that we will have six witnesses, who will be: Thomas Atcitty, who represents the New Mexico House of Representatives, who will discuss the Shiprock Hospital; Lydia Hubbard-Pourier, who will talk about Hantavirus; Norman Ration, who is the Acting Director of the Behavioral Health Services, Navajo Division of Health, and will talk about substance abuse; Peggy Nakai, who is the Health Program Manager, Navajo Division of Health, will talk about facilities; HIV/AIDS, Roselyn Chapela; and Environmental Health, Herman Shorty.

I would ask our witnesses to try to confine their statements to 5 minutes so that we will have plenty of time for questions and answers.

I was deeply alarmed when I learned of the President's budget proposal for Indian health care. The President's budget is calling for cutting the IHS budget by $247 million in 1995. When you eliminate the budget gimmicks, such as the assumption that the Indian Health Service will be able to collect $106 million in private health insurance, the budget cuts skyrocket to nearly $330 million.

Last year, the President assured Native Americans that his national health care plan would address their needs and concerns by expanding public health and prevention activities and to renovate and expand health clinics. Instead, this budget eliminates funding for new construction of hospitals, clinics and sanitation facilities, reduces funding for childhood immunizations, dental care and mental health programs, and calls for drastic staff reductions, nearly 2,000 over the next 2 years.

This budget is bitter medicine for Native Americans who continue to bear an increased burden of illness and premature mortality compared to other U.S. populations. It's especially troubling for the White Mountain Apache Tribe, which needs assistance to combat an alarming epidemic of suicide that has resulted in 14 deaths and 100 suicide attempts over a 13-month period.

President Zah captured the substance of tribal opinion when he said there is simply no logic or humanity in reducing health care services to those who so desperately need them, nor in expending millions of dollars to construct a needed hospital only to have it stand half vacant due to staff cuts. You have my pledge, that I'll do everything possible to reverse the budget cuts proposed in this budget.

I had longer remarks but I would like to abbreviate them because we would like to hear from Senator Domenici and our very long list of witnesses. Again, we welcome you here today and thank you for your participation with the witnesses, and thank you for your observance to the people who have come here. Thank you.

Now I would like to turn this microphone over to Senator Domenici.

STATEMENT OF HON. PETE V. DOMENICI, U.S. SENATOR FROM NEW MEXICO

Senator DOMENICI. Thank you very much, Senator McCain.

As you know, the Indian people are now represented in the U.S. Senate by the best committee in the history of the U.S. Senate. There is no doubt that Senator Dan Inouye, Senator John McCain, as chairman and vice chairman of that committee in the U.S. Senate, create the first committee that looks at Indian problems in a comprehensive way, and in a very real way have become very good advocates for the cause of the Indian people in our country, in New Mexico and Arizona and across this land.

Today we're here because there is a very, very serious problem. The problem of health care reform in this Nation and everybody anxiously awaits to see what the outcome of that will be. While on Indian country in particular here in Navajo country and more specifically right here at the new hospital, Indian health, instead of going forward, is going backward. Instead of providing much-needed services, living up to some commitments we've made, we're taking giant steps backward under the President's budget.

The President has been advised, early in January I advised him, shortly thereafter every single member of the Senate Committee on Indian Affairs of the United States wrote him a detailed letter which Senator McCain has just essentially explained. We have not had a commitment from the White House that that will be fixed, and all of us now are going to work together to see if we can get the Appropriations Committee in the U.S. Senate to take money from somewhere else in the budget of the United States.

Some of the areas that the President's asking for more money, we're going to have to take from them and put into Indian health just so we can keep pace with some basic commitments we have made, some real needs that are out here and across this land wherever Indian health is delivered by the Indian Health Service of the United States.

So all I can tell you is I want to hear again from the Indian people what they know about this pending disaster, and then to go back to Washington tomorrow and start the appropriations cycle with the full hope that with your support, with your push, with the Indian people in this instance demanding what is justly theirs, that we will in the next few months right this very serious budget problem for your people.

Thank you very much, and thank you, Senator, for inviting me and joining me in my State.

Senator McCAIN. Thank you very much, Senator Domenici, and again I would like to express my extreme pleasure and honor of working with you for so many years.

I would like to introduce our first witness, Congressman Jon Kyl, who has been very active on these issues, and as I mentioned, represents a significant portion of Navajo country in the Fourth Congressional District of Arizona. Welcome, Congressman Kyl.

STATEMENT OF HON. JON KYL, U.S. REPRESENTATIVE FROM ARIZONA

Mr. KYL. Thank you, Senator McCain and Senator Domenici, President Zah, Vice President Plummer. I appreciate the chance to join you and other members of the Senate Committee on Indian Affairs here today to examine the funding needs of the Indian Health Service.

Mr. Chairman, you will recall that I represented a large portion of the Navajo Nation before House district lines were redrawn in 1992. Although my district has changed, my concern about issues affecting the Navajo people has not, particularly with respect to health care. That is what brings me here today, to express my deep disappointment with the budget President Clinton has proposed for the IHS and the impact it will surely have on health care delivery for the Navajo people.

The President's fiscal year 1995 budget request, for example, includes enough funding to hire only about one-third of the staff necessary to fully staff and utilize the new Shiprock Hospital. It makes little sense to have invested so much in the construction of this facility only to have much of it idled by staff cuts now.

I would point out that this is not an area that is overserved. Waiting lists for care at IHS facilities are long. And people who are sick or injured often have to be transported on dirt roads up to 100 miles to receive care. Life expectancy among Navajos is well under the U.S. average. Infant deaths far exceed those of the overall U.S. population. This is an area of significant need.

Mr. Chairman, as the President of the Navajo Nation, Peterson Zah, wrote in a recent letter to me, and I'm quoting, "There is simply no logic in nor humanity in reducing health care services to those who so desperately need them." We need to set better priorities in the Congress. A fifth of the Health and Human Services Department staff cuts should not be borne by the IHS alone, as is proposed for 1995.

Health care should not be taken away from the very population that needs it most. Cutting Government spending does not have to mean across the board cuts or devastating cuts in the most important programs. It does mean rethinking priorities, eliminating the wasteful, obsolete or unnecessary programs, and putting off the luxuries for another day.

Mr. Chairman, I would like to submit for the record a copy of President Zah's letter, as well as letters from Genevieve Jackson and other tribal leaders in Arizona about the proposed budget cuts.

[Material to be inserted appears in appendix.]

Mr. KYL. I also look forward to working with you and my colleagues in the House for a budget that better reflects the needs of this community, and I thank you very much for holding this hearing.

Senator MCCAIN. Thank you, Congressman Kyl, and next we would like to hear from Peterson Zah, President of the Navajo Nation. Welcome, President Zah.

STATEMENT OF HON. PETERSON ZAH, PRESIDENT, NAVAJO NATION

President ZAH. Thank you.

Thank you, Senator, Representative Jon Kyl from the State of Arizona, then Genevieve Jackson, from the Navajo Nation Committee on Health and Social Services, Vice President Plummer, others that are at this hearing.

It was about perhaps 1 month ago that I contacted my good friend, Senator John McCain from Arizona, and explained to him what was being proposed, and that if those proposed budget cuts were to go through, I saw some problems that we as Navajo people and as Indian people were going to be greatly disappointed about, and that is the impact of those proposed reductions in FTEs.

And so I really wanted to thank both of you for coming today to have a first-hand look at the facility that is being built here, which is scheduled to be finished sometime this fall, but only to see that it's going to be half staffed. I don't think that the American public, the taxpayer, want to look at the facility over here and see it's going to be half empty. It's not going to be a very good public image for those taxpayers to see us spend so much money, over $35 million or $40 million, and then just to see it half empty for the next year. And we are extremely concerned about it.

During my lifetime, I have worked with the tribal government through probably four Presidents. And I'm extremely disappointed as to what's happening now. In the past there were some budget cuts, and we felt those budget cuts. But at the same time, we knew what the Nation was trying to do, and we understood some of the objectives that were being proposed by Congress. And we know that both of you are in a very particular situation with the budget cuts, and then there's also the needs of our Indian people and other people across America.

So we understand that. However, I'm extremely disappointed at what's happening now, the budget coming from the White House, for several reasons. One of them is that if you look at the proposed reduction in FTEs and then the proposed budget cut when it comes down to dollars, the OMB is taking a disproportionate share of the budget cuts on Indian programs rather than looking at all of the other programs, for example, within Health and Human Services.

And we are only asking for justice. We are only asking for fairness, and that these disparities should not really exist the way it is being proposed. And I know that you will do everything that you can within your power once you start the deliberation on the budget that you're going to try to restore as much of those as possible. And we from the Navajo Nation certainly appreciate that. And I just wanted to tell you about the seriousness of this proposal.

Again, we thank each of you for coming over, and we also thank the Congressman for coming to Shiprock Area and then having to look at, first-hand, the nice facilities that will be built here. And we would like to see that fully staffed so that we can take care of all of the health needs of the Navajo people.

I will recommend three things. One of them is that we request the assistance of Congress to waive the FTE reduction for Indian Health Service and to restore full funding to the Indian Health Service. Number two, we specifically request Congress to include funding for an additional 515 FTEs and activation costs for the Northern Navajo Medical Center. Third, we request Congress to make every effort to ensure that Indian Health Service budget is not further reduced.

In conclusion, there is no population in greater need of adequate health care than the American Indians. For generations, our people have lagged far behind the rest of America in every health category. This is unacceptable, especially in light of our special relationship with the United States, based on our treaties with the United States, and the Federal court decisions, Federal law and Presidential executive orders. This special relationship has been upheld as the law of the land.

The cuts and the reduction for Indian health flies in the face of this long history of law. The American Indian people gave up their lands and in return received the solemn promise of the United States that basic services such as health care would be provided to them.

The latest proposal to cut and reduce the Indian Health Service contradicts and violates this basic foundation of America's stand on government-to-government relationships between Indian tribes and the United States. If the proposed cuts go forward, we will not be able to handle this as something that we wanted to do all alone, and that is to provide quality health care.

The United States must be held accountable if it this is to happen. We will do whatever we need to do to make the United States fulfill its responsibility toward the Indian people.

Again, thank you for coming into Shiprock and then hearing from the Navajo people, which will be greatly impacted by these budget cuts. Thank you.

[Prepared statement of President Zah appears in appendix.]

Senator McCAIN. Thank you very much, President Zah, and your complete statement will be made part of the record, and thank you for a very strong statement.

Next we will hear from Genevieve Jackson, Councilwoman and Chairperson of the Health and Social Services Committee of the Navajo Tribal Council. We welcome you, Councilwoman Jackson.

STATEMENT OF GENEVIEVE JACKSON, COUNCILWOMAN AND CHAIRPERSON OF THE HEALTH AND SOCIAL SERVICES COMMITTEE, NAVAJO TRIBAL COUNCIL

Ms. JACKSON. Thank you, Senator McCain and Senator Domenici for coming to my humble community here in Shiprock, and the Honorable Jon Kyl that I'm presenting.

And I need to take my glasses off, I am unable to secure an appointment at the IHS, they are 3 or 4 months booked, so hopefully after this hearing the situation will change. [Laughter.]

My name is Genevieve Jackson, I am the Chairperson of the Health and Social Services Committee of the Navajo Nation Council, and also represent the Shiprock Chapter. There are several issues I would like to address today, all surrounding the topic of health care reform and its anticipated impact on Indian health programs in Arizona.

The Navajo Nation has been an active participant in the health care reform activities of the Clinton administration up until recently. We believed that the promises of this badly-needed reform will benefit Indian people, up until recently. The proposed FTE reduction plan that the Clinton administration has badly shaken our faith in the promises of health care reform.

The impact on health care to the people of the Navajo Nation will be devastating. The current figures are that almost 800 staff will be eliminated in one fiscal year, in addition to 150 positions projected for the new Northern Navajo Comprehensive Health Care Facility, formerly known as Shiprock Hospital, which were not funded for fiscal year 1995.

We are wondering whether our health care system will survive until health care reform measures are implemented. Let me highlight some facts about the Navajo Nation to help you understand the scenario we are facing. The Navajo Nation is the largest Indian reservation and the largest reservation-based Indian Tribe in the United States.

No. 2, the reservation land base is equal to the State of West Virginia and totals about 26,109 square miles. No. 3, organizationally the Navajo Area has 8 service units, 6 hospitals, with a total of 390 beds, 8 health centers and 14 health stations. Senators and visitors, non-Indian visitors to the Navajo Nation, beware, do not become sick or be in an accident while you are in Navajo Nation. All the beds may be taken.

[Applause.]

Ms. JACKSON. No. 4, the fiscal year 1993 user population is 230,255. This encompasses almost 20 percent of the total Indian population and is growing at an estimated rate of 2 to 3 percent per year. No. 5, the median age of the population on Navajo is 21.6 compared to 33 years for the general U.S. population. No. 6, about 50 percent of the population is age 19 and younger. No. 7, the per capita income of the Navajo Nation is $4,108, very low in comparison to the U.S. population.

The median family income is also $10,433, again, substantially lower than the U.S. median family income of $30,056. Fifty-eight percent of individuals on the Navajo Nation have incomes below the poverty level. These figures are based on the 1999 U.S. census reports. No. 8, the Navajo Area IHS budget is $200 million, or 10.5 percent of the total IHS budget.

No. 9, Navajo Area IHS has 22.9 percent of total IHS staffing, or a total of 3,200 staff. No. 10, Navajo has continued to account for about 27 percent of the in-patient workload for all of IHS, and for about 20 percent of all the outpatient visits in all IHS facilities.

Number 11, the average level of need funded for Navajo Area in fiscal year 1992 was 67 percent, including Medicaid and Medicare collections. The level of need funded is derived at by showing what percent of ideal funding we are currently at. That is, by dividing our available resource by what resources we should ideally have.

Our experience has been that IHS by policy only funds Indian Health Service at a level less than 85 percent defined level of need funded. In fiscal year 1993, M&M collections rose to a level of $39 million. These were additional resources the Navajo Area is providing and is increasing at 15 percent a year. The figure is in addition to the Congressional appropriations we receive.

Number 12, the Navajo Area has many unmet health needs, similar to other tribes and areas nationwide. Basic quality ambulatory care is provided to Navajo patients, but waiting times are frustratingly long, and it often takes 1 month or more to get an appointment in a specialty clinic.

Such basic services such as general care are not easy to obtain, and long appointment lists and waiting times are common. Many specialty services are not available at local clinics or hospitals and oftentimes Navajo patients are referred 200 or 300 miles to the nearest non-IHS medical facility that offers specialty services. Lack of sanitation and plumbing in 15 percent of homes also has a serious effect on health services.

Manpower is attributable to the success of collecting third-party resources. With the FTE ceiling in place now, we are not able to be as aggressive as we were in the past.

These dollars should not be used to offset our budget. We do not want the third-party resources to be used as penalties against Federal appropriations that we would have otherwise received. In terms of the total FTE cuts, 252 FTEs would be eliminated, and all 324 funded vacant positions would not be filled. Over 80 percent of these positions are doctors and nurses for people who are delivering health care services. This, Senators, is unacceptable.

Another area in which we are being adversely affected is by the senior level ceiling on GS–14 and GS–15 positions. The ceiling that is imposed on us also penalizes doctors, limits our ability to hire new doctors and limit promotions to 20 positions, intern to senior level positions. It is absolutely impossible to implement the proposed personnel reductions without drastically impacting the health care of Navajo people and Native Americans in general. Without some relief from Congress or the Clinton administration, the only option at this point appears to be a reduction in force, RIF, which has been officially requested by the IHS.

How can this gloomy picture be consistent with the bright promise of health care reform? It isn't. We keep thinking that someone has made a serious mistake through poor planning or sheer ignorance. But who? I don't know. But Indian people are sure to suffer as a result.

The Navajo Nation recognizes that health care costs are rising at an alarming rate, and that all American citizens are entitled to a comprehensive package of health care benefits. Indian Health Service has provided health care to Native Americans throughout the years in fulfillment of trust and treaty obligations. During their Congressional review of the proposed Health Security Act and current health reform, the Federal Government's responsibility to continue providing health care, education and other services to American Indians and Alaska Natives must prevail. The government-to-government relationship between Native American tribes, including the Navajo Nation and the Federal Government, must be sustained.

There is an irony to this situation that I must point out. On one hand, the U.S. Government has obligations to provide a comprehensive array of health services to Native people. The health care reform proposal aims to provide a comprehensive health care benefits package to all Americans. Yet on the other hand, FTE reductions are being imposed on IHS, the primary health care provider in Indian Country. How can the Navajo Nation embrace these perhaps well-intentioned yet conflicting initiatives?

Indian Health Service has a transition period of 5 years. That is to 1999. To bring its resources up to par in order to provide the comprehensive benefits package promised in the health care proposals, by no means will the Navajo Area IHS and the Navajo Nation be able to obtain the idea scenario under health care reform without additional resources.

Currently, we are still trying to bring the health care system on Navajo up to a level comparable with the rest of the U.S. and literally quantum leaps would be needed to offer a true, comprehensive set of health care benefits to the Navajo people.

Thank you for allowing me this opportunity to voice my views. Also, if you will indulge, I am the Chairperson of the Child Sexual Abuse program on the Navajo Nation, so I will also give that testimony.

In August 1990, a multi-agency Navajo Nation ad hoc committee on child sexual abuse was organized to seek ways for improving the response of existing organizations to child sexual abuse and neglect cases on the Navajo Nation. In August 1992, the Navajo Nation Child Protect Team emerged with a CAC, which is the Child Advocacy Committee.

The CAC has dual roles, of No. 1, being an oversight body for the local child protection teams on the Navajo Nation, and No. 2, serving as an advisory and advocacy body for the Navajo Child Sexual Abuse Program. The CAC is compromised of multidisciplinary professionals which coordinate preventive and protective services for Navajo child abuse victims and their families on the Navajo Nation. CAC seeks continual acknowledgement, support and cooperation from all entities involved in this program.

In October 1990, Congress earmarked funding in the fiscal year 1991 Interior appropriations for the Child Advocacy Committee. In the spring of 1990, the ad hoc committee completed the development of a comprehensive 5-year plan to enable the Navajo Nation and other organizations to make incremental steps, year by year, in addressing child abuse issues starting in 1991 and ending in 1996. The ad hoc committee identified Navajo Child Sexual Abuse Program demonstration sites of Tuba City and Fort Defiance, AZ and Shiprock, NM, to begin in the fall of 1990.

However, due to funding misappropriation at the area level, Navajo Child Sexual Abuse Project was not able to provide services until September 1991. At the beginning of fiscal year 1992–93, NCSAP was unsuccessful in hiring qualified specialists for the three treatment teams. Late in fiscal year 1992, Tuba City Child Advocacy Committee hired its treatment team. At the end of fiscal year 1992, Fort Defiance and Shiprock hired treatment team members.

Hence, fiscal year 1992 was the first full year of operations for the three treatment teams. The Navajo Nation also appropriated general funds to establish NCSAP in Crown Point, NM and Chimney, AZ. Because the symptoms and causes of child sexual abuse and neglect are multifaceted, treatment and prevention must be comprehensive and multidisciplinary. Victims of severe cases of child sexual abuse and neglect require long-term care and services.

The NCSAP provides treatment services that are holistic and customized to the needs of Navajo clientele. The NCSAP also implements a multidisciplinary response to child sexual abuse and neglect cases which involve a variety of human services professionals, such as social workers, Navajo traditional counselors, mental health specialists, prosecutors, criminal investigators, attorneys and law enforcement officials and the FBI.

The Navajo Nation provides the following recommendations. No. 1, the Navajo Nation recommends that Federal funds for the Navajo Child Sexual Abuse Project and other child abuse related programs are reoccurring, so that current initiatives within the program are developed and approved. The Navajo Nation would like to continue providing and improving intervention treatment and prevention services to Navajo child abuse victims and their families in a timely and efficient manner.

No. 2, in order to avoid further funding problems of the Navajo Child Sexual Abuse Project, moneys at the agency level, the Navajo Nation recommends that the NCSAP have a central office in Window Rock, AZ to receive Federal appropriations directly from the Federal resources, instead of the current process of receiving funding from the BIA and IHS or other agencies. The NCSAP did not really develop until the third year of funding because of miscommunication and problems with the Federal agencies disbursing the funding in the first and second year.

No. 3, the Navajo Nation urges Congress and the Administration to provide full funding for Public Law 101-630, the Indian Child Protection and Family Violence Act. We are disappointed that the administration did not request any funding for Public Law 101-630 in the fiscal year 1995 budget, and never has appropriated any money for the act since the enactment of Public Law 101-630.

No. 4, the Navajo Nation requests Congress and the administration to require the BIA boarding school child protection team to participate and be a part of the local community child protection teams and multidisciplinary teams for comprehensive services for child abuse victims across the Navajo Nation.

The Navajo Nation appreciates and thanks Senators McCain, Domenici, and Congressman Kyl for their support in advocating comprehensive child abuse services to Navajo children. Without your support, Senators, for the Navajo Child Sexual Abuse Project, the majority of our Navajo clientele would not have received treatment services. And I would also like to add, the Navajo Nation has proclaimed April as the Prevention of Child Abuse and Prevention of Child Sexual Abuse Month for the Navajo Nation.

Thank you very much.

[Prepared statement of Ms. Jackson appears in appendix.]

Senator McCain. Thank you very much, Ms. Jackson, for a very strong and compelling statement.

I would like to now ask Marshall Plummer, the Vice President of the Navajo Nation, for his remarks.

STATEMENT OF MARSHALL PLUMMER, VICE PRESIDENT, NAVAJO NATION

Mr. Plummer. Thank you, Senator.

Senator Domenici and myself would like to welcome you Arizonians.

[Applause.]

Mr. Plummer. There are a couple of things I would like to touch upon, I know President Zah touched upon certain points, and I would like to be more specific in some of these areas in addition to what Councilwoman Jackson had to say.

I think the two things that we kind of have common interest in is one, that through your many years of service, including the Congressman, many years of service, you have put in place some foundations that will help Indian nations. Our interest should be to protect those foundations. And what is resulting, based on the Federal cutbacks, whether it be the Indian Health Service or BIA, we're finding that a lot of that is being dismantled. And I would like to join with the Senators and of course the Congressman in assuring ourselves that we will sit together and protect those interests.

Second, in regards to the comments made by President Zah and of course by Councilwoman Jackson regarding treaty obligations, an analogy can be made wherein I go purchase a vehicle, and I sign a contract, and a treaty is basically a contract. Now, if I'm not paying on that particular vehicle, if I get behind, I guarantee you, the company that sold me that particular vehicle will be here in a couple of months and load that vehicle up and take it away from me.

I think that the President of the United States and those that are now beginning to acquaint themselves with Indian issues need to be made aware of the simple fact that there is a contract in place and if the U.S. Government does not fulfill its obligations, we are ready then to reassume those lands which we gave up.

[Applause.]

Mr. PLUMMER. Senator, Congressman, we would only ask that we get some assurance, assurances from the Federal Government that the services will continue, instead of penalizing the Indian Health Service. They ought to use the Indian Health Service as a model for the rest of America. When you're talking about social medicine, that's essentially what's happening through this health care reform at the present time. The Indian Health Service has been in practice for many years. And I think that one can capitalize on that and improve the service of health services. I think maybe that could even be put forth as a recommendation to your fellow Senators and Congressmen there in Washington.

To be more specific on some of the things that I said that we need to protect, a good example is I know Senator Domenici and Senator McCain, you've been involved in getting the infrastructure on Indian reservations, for getting loan programs such as housing, HUD programs, all of those things are great for Indian Country. The problem is that we've been made aware now that the 86–101 projects, I understand, which was slated for $23 million for Navajo alone, has not been included in the executive budget. And what that does, it slows everything down. You can build a house, but if you don't put in water, it isn't going to do you any good.

And so those types of things, you've done certain things, but in order to make it a full package, what's happened is that the executive branch has decided to cut those funding categories. Landfills, regulations have put now a tremendous burden on communities and in particular Indian reservations, knowing that one landfill probably costs $10 million just to set up. We're going to need a lot of help in setting those up in this nation of ours.

The fact that President Zah mentioned the Shiprock Hospital, there is also another facility south of here, at Tohatchi, a brand-new facility, and it's my understanding that there are 63 physicians that are slated now to be deleted. We're talking about approximately $3.3 million which we would like to have restored to have fully staffed that Tohatchi clinic.

In addition to that, the Gallup Hospital, I understand, is also going to be renovated, which will then most likely have patients that will be referred over to the Tohatchi clinic, because the Gallup Hospital is not supposed to be in full operation. In addition to that, Senators and Congressman, we have worked hard to set priorities for Navajo, new construction of hospitals and clinics.

And as you see now at Shiprock and also Tohatchi, there are other facilities such as Caliente, and also the Winslow Hospital, that are slated. Now, if IHS is going to take a cut, we're not going to see those facilities, and that's all your work going down the drain, and I know that you don't want that.

So we're calling upon you to join hands with us, and I think that's the only way that we're going to be able to overcome what is before us.

One other item that I would like to thank Senator Domenici on is the Trading With Indians Act. We've got three or four Navajo individuals who are now beginning to run businesses. And this law, as I understand, was instituted in the thirties and still stands today. And it's a stupid law, and we need to get rid of that.

[Applause.]

Mr. PLUMMER. Congressman, I would like to call upon you, and I understand now it's before the House, I'm not sure which particular committee, but we're going to need some leverage to get that through. And I know the Senators have done their job and it's gone through the Senate, but we really are going to need your assistance as far as this particular package.

I would like to just close with a couple of inquiries, or ask that there be followup on this project that has been set in place for Navajo, the uranium miller's State exemption. Senator Bingaman introduced that and got $500,000. We would like to ask for your assistance to see if we can get that money to us as soon as possible.

Of course, some of the work that's been done by President Zah and others, Michael Begaye and others on the radiation exposure compensation, I understand there is no money slated for this year, and I would like to have an inquiry and see if we can get additional moneys set in place for this.

I want to personally thank the three of you for being here with us today. This shows the commitment that you have to the Navajo people. Thank you.

Senator MCCAIN. Thank you very much, Vice President Plummer.

And now I would like to hear from Judy Knight-Frank, the Chairperson of the Ute Mountain Ute Tribe. Thank you for being with us this morning, Chairperson Frank.

STATEMENT OF JUDY KNIGHT-FRANK, CHAIRMAN, UTE MOUNTAIN UTE TRIBE

Ms. FRANK. Thank you very much.

Our reservation is the New Mexico-Colorado boundary. I'm here because we also go into New Mexico, we have some townships just north of the San Juan coal plant. We also go into the State of Utah. Our small clinic is located in Colorado, in Towaoc, Colorado. We have a population of 1,850 people.

According to our records, we have over 8,000 records, our small clinic does service a lot of the Navajo population, which at times leaves our people without services. We do utilize the Cortez Hospital, but that's under contract services. I believe that some of the Navajo people are also utilizing our contract services there.

But we're a very small tribe compared to Navajo. But we need services just like everybody else, and we do use the hospital that is available here in Shiprock. But because of the waiting, because of the beds being full, because of not having physicians, pediatricians and other professionals that are not there full time, we have to go to contract services.

We have supported building this hospital, and we were very disappointed when we heard that the positions were going to be cut, because we still need the beds, we need the services more than ever, because I believe that our Indian population is growing, not only Indian but all nations. So the hospital is really needed, and we support the building of it.

We would also like to request at this time if at all possible that we be given *x* number of beds. We have the supporting documents. The reason for that is that when we send patients down here, the beds are full and our people have to be sent elsewhere. That's where the contract moneys come in.

The Ute Mountain Tribe has available Blue Cross/Blue Cross for the tribal employees. What we have found in the years we have had it, that IHS has to do third party billings. This year, we had to go to another health plan. What we found is that now that IHS is not considered a prime care provider, they cannot be paid for third party billings. I asked the health director why that was, and he said it has to do with IHS regulations not being able to bill Indian tribes.

I'm letting you know today that there is a problem there. We have tried to get our employees to take on family coverage. That is about $480 a month. Our people don't make money to cover that kind of coverage for their families. Therefore, IHS is where they go to get health coverage. We try to get our people to understand that these things are necessary, but they know that we have a treaty with the United States, and there are certain services that are supposed to given to us in return for all that we gave up

So today, I would ask the Senators here that the cuts not be taken, that because it affects our small tribe, and we are in the Southern Colorado service unit, I think there are four positions being cut. That's such a small margin compared to what's being proposed on Navajo, but when we have one full-time doctor and one part-time and one dentist, you know, that's a lot. We can't afford to lose those.

And those people that I have mentioned, the Navajo Nation does provide, they do utilize those clinics. So if we have any more cuts, this is going to be a hardship, both on the Ute Mountain Ute Tribe and on the Navajo Nation. Our dentist, it's the same, we have one dentist. And I know that a lot of people in the surrounding area do utilize that.

There is attached to this statement a list that shows where people come from. They come from as far away as Albuquerque, NM; Chinile, AZ; Crown Point, AZ; Kagenta, AZ; Tuba City, AZ; and Gallup, NM. We know there are dentists in those areas. Why do they come to where we're at? Maybe the waiting is not so long.

But our people, when they're in need of medical services and go to our small clinic, the Ute Mountain Ute people, many of them will not wait and they will do without services. So we are providing services to, the Navajo Nation and to the Ute Mountain Utes, but in many ways we're not giving the full services that our people, the Ute Mountain Utes, need.

So these reductions do affect all Indian nations, and that is why I'm here today, because we are very opposed to the cuts and we have supported this hospital. I have also done some research and gone back through old records. The Ute Mountain Tribe had requested a hospital, a 25-bed hospital, back in the seventies, which was not built because there are rules that say if you have a hospital within a certain mile radius that's not feasible.

So we have tried to do what we can, but we would appreciate the Senators that are here today, if you would do whatever you can so that these cuts will not take place. And I thank you for the opportunity to be here, and I thank you for the support that you give Indian tribes and the committees that you serve on, and it's very well appreciated by my people. Thank you again.

[Prepared statement of Ms. Knight-Frank appears in appendix.]

Senator McCAIN. Thank you very much, Chairperson Knight-Frank.

Out of curiosity, Chairperson Knight-Frank, how far did you come today to come to the hearing this morning?

Ms. KNIGHT-FRANK. It was 25 miles.

Senator McCAIN. Thank you.

Mr. President, did you have any additional comments before we close this down?

President ZAH. Senator, thank you.

One of the things that sometimes we as Indian people have a tendency to overlook is the employment of the Indian people, for example, on your committee. We have at this meeting with us three or four Indian people that work with the U.S. Senate Committee on Indian Affairs, and I want you to know that we really appreciate the fact that you employ them. Because if anyone knows these issues first-hand, it's them. And I would like for the three of them to stand and be recognized by the audience.

Dan Lewis is a Navajo from Navajo Nation here in Window Rock, and we really, really appreciate your coming with both of the Senators, and then be their eyes and ears.

[Applause.]

President ZAH. So we really appreciate that.

The other thing is that there are some school facilities out there on the Navajo that are really run down. And I know that I wanted to give you a copy of the proposal that I think we also need to take a look at within the Department of the Interior. Their budget is also being considered for cutting.

And I come from a place called Low Mountain, it's God's country, it's a heaven for us, and we have a little, tiny school out there. The roof is coming down, every time it rains, the water comes down into the classroom. The kids are just having a tough time, and they're ready to close down that school. The Indian Health Service and the health people are saying, "If you don't do anything about this, we may just close down the school, you may have to send your kids elsewhere."

And that really needs your attention when you look at the Department of the Interior budget. So I would like to also for the record submit a proposal that they put together to this committee for your consideration.

Again, thank you.

Senator McCain. Thank you very much, Mr. President.

I would mention the other two members of our staff who are here, Diane Humetewa. Diane, would you stand? She's a Hopi.

[Applause.]

Senator McCain. And Eleanor McComber, who's of the Mohawk Tribe. Eleanor, thank you for being with us.

[Applause.]

Senator McCain. And Dan Lewis' parents are here, sitting behind us, who are obviously proud of their son, as he is of them.

[Applause.]

Senator McCain. I would like to thank the panel, and I would like to ask Senator Domenici if he has any questions for this panel.

Senator Domenici. I just wanted to ask Genevieve, you said that you had Blue Cross Coverage. Not Genevieve, excuse me, Judy. You said you had some, and do I understand that it used to apply and doesn't or is this a new thing?

Ms. Knight-Frank. We have Prime Care Blue Cross, it's another portion of Blue Cross, but what we have found is, we had to change, we had to shop around for another insurance because our rates went up 38 percent. We just could not afford that. So we had to find the best rate we could find. And that had not been a problem before. But this other coverage that we have will not recognize IHS as the prime care provider. They will not recognize most sub-doctors as prime care providers.

So at this point, I don't know what we're going to do. I think we were getting some money from Blue Cross before. We're not going to be getting that any more. But they say it is an IHS regulation.

Senator Domenici. I understand. We'll look into that. Thank you.

Senator McCain. Thank you very much to this panel. I want to thank you for your contributions, and we look forward to continuing our efforts together. We're in agreement as to what the problem is, and we're in agreement as to what needs to be done. We also will, I think, be helped by the following witnesses and obtaining a good knowledge base of what needs to be done.

I thank this fine panel, thank you very much for being with us.

I would like to ask John Hubbard, who is the Director of the Navajo Area Indian Health Service, to join us. Mr. Hubbard.

And while Mr. Hubbard is testifying, I would be glad to have the next panel come and sit behind him, so we can move forward as quickly as possible. Thomas Atcitty; Lydia Hubbard-Pourier; Norman Ration; Peggy Nakai; Roselyn Chapela; and Herman Shorty. If you would come and sit behind him so we could move right into the next one.

Mr. Hubbard, we would be glad to hear your prepared statement or remarks you would like to make. We will make your complete statement a part of the record, and welcome, and please proceed. And would you do me the favor, for the record, is it correct, you're accompanied by Dr. Doug Peter and Dr. Allen Craig, is that who's with you this morning?

Mr. Hubbard. I have Dr. Allen Craig, our Clinical Director, who's here with me today.

Senator McCain. Thank you.

Mr. Hubbard, please proceed.

STATEMENT OF JOHN HUBBARD, DIRECTOR, NAVAJO AREA INDIAN HEALTH SERVICE, ACCOMPANIED BY DR. ALLEN CRAIG, M.D., CLINICAL DIRECTOR, SHIPROCK HOSPITAL

Mr. HUBBARD. Thank you, Senator McCain, Senator Domenici, Congressman Kyl. I want to welcome you also to Shiprock, NM, to hear testimony on IHS issues. I'm here today with Dr. Allen Craig, our clinical director of the Shiprock Hospital here. He doesn't have a statement but if there are questions, clinical questions, he will be responding to those. Some of the issues have already been addressed today, and in the interest of time I will briefly highlight my prepared statement.

Organizationally, IHS in the Navajo Area has 8 service units. We operate 6 hospitals with a total of 390 beds. The fiscal year 1994 user population for us in Navajo is 230,255. Health care is a labor-intensive business. The Navajo Area has about 23 percent of all of the Indian Health Service's staffing. Our staffing total is about 3,500. This figure represents Federal employment, and does not take into account tribally-operated programs in other areas.

The Navajo Area submitted a proposed FTE reduction plan to IHS headquarters in response to the current administration's initiative to reduce the number of employees in the Federal Government. The plan has not been approved to date. Target goals for the Navajo Area were FTE levels of 3,041 FTEs for the current fiscal year and 2,977 for September 1995. I want to stress that the planning for FTEs is just that, it's planning and has not been approved yet.

Appropriations for the Navajo Child Sexual Abuse Program have been provided to Navajo Area and the Bureau of Indian Affairs since 1990. Of $798,000 allocated to Navajo, $298,000 is IHS funds awarded to the tribe, the rest are funneled through the BIA. In 1994, IHS and BIA joined in developing a special task force to address the issue of child abuse and other dysfunctional behavior, especially in the boarding school segment.

Another major activity for Navajo Area IHS staff is the implementation of the Navajo Nation's comprehensive 5-year plan on child abuse and neglect.

While the problem of AIDS and HIV infection continues to increase among Navajo people, Centers for Disease Control and Prevention resources allocated to Navajo have decreased. The first HIV case on Navajo appeared in 1982. Since then, care has been provided to 49 HIV positive and persons with AIDS at PHS hospitals here on Navajo, of which 17 have died. AIDS victims represent all ages and both sexes. Transmission among Navajo people has been by each of the known pathways.

Ambulance service training, orientation and other continuing education opportunities are provided on care and maintenance of HIV-affected patients. Much attention is given to worker protection issues to control transmission of HIV in occupational procedures.

Here in Shiprock, we have the Four-Corners Regional Adolescent Treatment Center. It is fully accredited with the JCAHO since 1992. The facility is one of the nine operating in the United States and is among those mandated by Public Law 99-570. It has 24 beds for a 90-day program for adolescent Native Americans. Recently, the Navajo Nation and the Indian Health Service have developed a Regional Resource Directory. It was published and disseminated to over 200 organizations. It will be updated in the very near future.

The Navajo Nation and the Navajo Area IHS as you know experienced a devastating new illness called the Hantavirus in the spring and summer of 1993. To date, a total of 67 persons have been affected nationwide. There have been 29 Native Americas affected, 17 of whom have died. Of these, 22 were Navajo, including 12 deaths. Though Hantavirus Pulmonary Syndrome has had a nationwide impact, the vast majority of cases have been located in the southwestern United States.

Public education and training remains the major thrust of our efforts, the disease is preventable. Navajo Area IHS and the Navajo Nation have been instrumental in the ongoing effort to inform area residents of the dangers of exposures and methods to avoid contracting the disease, especially in the springtime, when most of us begin spring cleaning activities.

The annual funding for Public Law 86–121, The Indian Sanitation Facilities Construction Act of 1959, has been in the range of $85 million annually, and because of its huge need, the Navajo Area has received over 24 percent of this total funding. The Navajo Housing Authority provides funds to install outside utility for numerous HUD housing sites, and the Navajo-Hopi Indian Relocation Commission provides funding to serve Navajo Relocatee housing sites. Matching funds from the Navajo Nation's Capital Improvement Program and Community development Block Grant programs also augment the projects. So the lack of these dollars not only give us less funds, but eliminates additional funds—from these sources—that have added to the construction of these projects.

Presently, the Navajo Area, the Navajo Nation and the BIA are in the process of finalizing a Memorandum of Agreement which will define the role of these entities for the inventory and remediation of non-permitted solid waste disposal sites, or open dumps, here on the Navajo Nation. At this time, the MOU is proceeding through the Navajo Nation government. Once it's signed, we will proceed with implementing the agreement. The MOU calls for the three entities to prioritize sites for closure, formulate remediation plans and assure the development of alternative solid waste management systems.

This concludes our remarks, and we will be happy to answer any questions. Thank you very much.

Senator McCain. Thank you very much, Mr. Hubbard.

Dr. Craig, would you give the committee a brief assessment of these reductions are not reversed, just give us an overall picture if you could in a few words as to what the impact is going to cost on your ability to provide the much- needed services for Native Americans at your hospital.

Dr. Craig. I think the FTE reductions, if implemented at Shiprock in particular, will have an impact on the care we're able to provide. Our staff is working very hard as it is, and I think that the FTE they're proposing at Shiprock is approximately 95. As Mr. Hubbard said, these have not been approved by headquarters and not been implemented yet. But they're proposing to reduce our staff by 95 over the next year and a half, approximately. I think this will increase the amount of time patients have to wait for appointments.

Senator McCain. Roughly what would that increase be, just as a rough estimate, in patient delay?

Dr. Craig. I guess the delay would probably increase by 30 to 60 days in terms of getting elective appointments.

Senator McCain. A delay of 30 to 60 days in order to get an appointment?

Dr. Craig. Yes; beyond what it is now. Now it's often 30 to 60 days, currently, so it will probably double the waiting time.

Senator McCain. So someone could wait as long as 4 months in order to get an appointment?

Dr. Craig. That could possibly occur, yes.

Senator McCain. Thank you. Please proceed. Is there anything else you would like to add?

Dr. Craig. I think the other concern we have is a budgetary concern that relates to the FTE reduction. Right now at Shiprock we're projecting a deficit of approximately $3 million in this fiscal year, and next year, if our funding does not increase, that will certainly increase with inflation and expenses related to operating the new hospital.

So there will be a double effect, the FTE reductions will affect our ability to provide care and our budgetary constraints will make it difficult, as well.

Senator McCain. Dr. Craig it's my understanding that the staffing level would be at about 54 percent, is that correct, of the hospital, if these reductions were enacted?

Dr. Craig. In terms of the projections for the new hospital?

Senator McCain. Yes.

Dr. Craig. Yes; that's correct.

Senator McCain. Would that mean that you would just shut down portions of the hospital?

Dr. Craig. We anticipate we will be able to provide less services. We would not be able to operate all 75 beds in the new hospital. We would only be able to operate two of the five operating rooms in the new hospital. In effect, it may have a more significant impact than that, because of the medical inflation and the increasing deficit, we may not be able to provide the level of services we currently provide.

Senator McCain. So what happens to these people?

Dr. Craig. For the most part, these patients will have to wait longer for elective surgery, elective procedures, and outpatient visits. If it's an emergency, the patients will have to be sent out to other facilities, and use contract health services funds for that.

Senator McCain. And that, of course the contract health services would be very expensive. Do you know how much that would be?

Dr. Craig. We're spending an average of approximately $6 million at Shiprock each year in contract health services dollars in the last 1 or 2 years. I don't know the exact numbers. I would anticipate it would increase substantially. And actually, we're a little bit concerned that we're going to run out of contract health services dollars this fiscal year anyway. So I'm not sure what next year holds. We're very concerned about that.

Senator McCAIN. Thank you. Finally, Mr. Hubbard, you're the messenger, and we're not trying to shoot you. Unfortunately, you don't make policy. I'm sure that if you did make policy, you would not advocate such reductions as these, and you don't have to respond to that.

I would like to point out that thanks to the efforts of my colleague from New Mexico, President Zah, and many others, there has been a letter sent to the Director of the Office of Management and Budget, and for the benefit of our friends here, the Office of Management and Budget is basically the one that has got the final decision making authority and I'm happy to note that the Secretary of Health and Human Services, in response to a letter from nine of us that Senator Domenici was responsible for, has requested that the Office of Management and Budget give a waiver on these reductions of FTEs.

Now, we haven't got an answer from the Office of Management and Budget, but at least we are getting some people's attention and I'm appreciative of that, and Mr. Hubbard, I'm appreciative of your recommendations that these decisions be reversed. The bad news is, we have no request for the restoration of the proposed budget cuts, but we'll work on that as well. So thank you for being here.

Senator Domenici.

Senator DOMENICI. I just want to say to Mr. Hubbard, I think you handled the Hantavirus situation very well, the region did, Indian Health did. Obviously, it's a very, very difficult problem. I was up here with you all and with the doctors. I'm very hopeful that the extra research money that went into the U.S. Government's research facilities will continue and that we will find soon some of the mysteries behind it, and Doctor, I know you're concerned about it. Everybody in Navajo Country is. It is not exclusively just part of America's problem, but clearly our Navajo people need to know as much as we can give them about how to protect themselves, and I hope that's going on and taking place.

Could you just tell me what you think about it, whether people are informed about what they should and shouldn't do regarding this virus?

Mr. HUBBARD. I think for the most part they are. There has been an intensive campaign to educate the people about the dangers of rodents. However, there is much more work to be done in this area. The Navajo Nation really has been aggressive in getting the word out through various means. There was a hotline that was established and the work that's going on today I think really has helped in not having any more cases. And we appreciate your comments.

Senator DOMENICI. Mr. Chairman, I just want to say with reference to Shiprock Hospital and people in this area that have been for so long patient, and on the other hand expecting something very important to happen in their lives with this facility, I shared all of that with you. It's taken us almost longer than one would believe to get that hospital under construction and finally get it built. I tell you, I am really embarrassed. I am embarrassed for the United States of America to build this facility——

[Applause.]

Senator DOMENICI. [continuing]. To build this facility and then have you have to come here, and it's not your fault, and tell us that it will only be 54 percent utilized when the people of this Navajo Nation cry out for just fairness in health care, and we're going to have this beautiful facility that any place, anywhere in the world, would love to have, and we can't even open it.

So we're going to do what we can, and we want you to understand that we don't know how this policy was made. If we get another chance, maybe we'll ask the President to take another look. He's corresponded with us and thus far it seems like he's being told that everything's going to come out all right. In fact, I don't know who's advising him. I have a letter from him that clearly his advisors don't even understand what's going on here, from what I can tell.

So obviously, maybe he doesn't yet understand what's going on, and I hope that's the case, so we might get him to help us. It would be a lot easier to change his budget, he can still do that, and took money from somewhere else and put it here, then we won't have to struggle with other committees to try to take their money to put in this program. Thanks, Mr. Chairman.

Mr. KYL. Thank you. I would like to just second what both of the Senators have said, and ask either one of you just one question. It's my understanding that there have already been some preliminary meetings to discuss what might have to happen in the way of cutbacks on services if we can't get this reversed. Perhaps I shouldn't be getting too specific here, but is it correct, for example, that you might not be able to keep the intensive care unit open in the event that this funding situation shouldn't be reversed? Is that one of the possibilities?

Dr. PETER. We've actually spent the last 2 days with our governing body members in Shiprock to discuss different scenarios in terms of FTE reductions and being fully funded for the new hospital and not having any additional funds. And certainly, closing the intensive care unit is one of the options we discussed, among many others.

Mr. KYL. Thank you. That would be a very, very difficult situation, and I think all of us want to ensure that that doesn't happen.

Thank you.

Senator MCCAIN. Thank you very much.

Instead of having all six, since it's a small table, perhaps we'll just take the first three, if that's agreeable, and then we'll take the following three after that. And of course, our first witness would be Thomas Atcitty. He is a member of the New Mexico House of Representatives. Lydia Hubbard-Pourier, who is the Executive Director of the Navajo Division of Health, on the issue of Hantavirus, and Norman Ration, who is the Acting Director of the Department of Behavioral Health, who has testified before our committee on previous occasions. Welcome back, sir.

Representative Atcitty, thank you for being with us today. I'm sure you've taken time from your otherwise very busy schedule and we thank you. Please proceed.

STATEMENT OF THOMAS ATCITTY, MEMBER, NEW MEXICO HOUSE OF REPRESENTATIVES

Mr. ATCITTY. Thank you, Mr. Chairman.

In fact, I was in Santa Fe this morning, and hurried back for this important meeting. This has been one my projects for the past few years, the hospital. Over 20 years ago, we had this hospital designed, and the plans sat for 20 years, the model sat around gathering dust. And so we started again a few years ago.

Mr. Chairman, Senator Domenici, Congressman Kyl, President Zah and the panel members, and all those community members that are interested in the project here, thank you for offering the Shiprock Hospital Steering Committee this opportunity to testify on the need for additional staffing for the new Shiprock Hospital and the impact of the FTE reduction.

I do not need to educate you on the importance of quality health care services for the Navajo people. You acknowledged our need for a new hospital in Shiprock by appropriating $53 million for the planning, design and construction of a replacement facility in fiscal year 1987, 1992, and 1993. Unfortunately, the President's fiscal year 1995 budget does not contain any moneys to fully staff and operate the new Northern Navajo Medical Center.

At Shiprock, we have four times as many patients per doctor as the national ratio. The 515 new positions will include a ratio and make it easier for our people to see, as much as possible, the same doctors, and receive sufficient time for a thorough examination. But any increase in the number of providers requires an additional increase in support staff. Without any new nurses and support staff we can forget about our plans for new specialty services such as specialized surgery, ophthalmology, urology, ear, nose, and throat.

If we cannot increase out staff, how will our facility be maintained? Who will operate the much-needed medical equipment that will be provided, such as our CT scanners? If our x ray technicians are assisting with CT scans, routine diagnostics, x rays, ultrasonic tests will have to be deferred. Or, do we not use a scanner and refer patients to outside hospitals, which is very expensive? How will we keep up with our increasing medical needs, such as diabetes, high blood pressure, heart disease, and the growing needs of our families and communities?

Decisions that only focus on direct medical care are a threat to our community health programs. We have a commitment to all our people in the community, reaching out to public health, nursing, environmental health programs, emotional health and disease prevention. Our programs for immunizations, adolescent services and women's health have received national recognition. In Shiprock, 95 percent of our children are immunized because IHS and tribal programs work together with families.

No matter what decisions are made on staffing and funding, it is clear that the health needs of our Navajo people will not go away, and will need to be met somehow. For the past 10 years, specialized medical services provided by IHS were recognized by Congress and exempted from Federal ceilings on full-time equivalent positions.

In fiscal year 1994, the exemption was rescinded, and IHS was included in the ceilings and in fact instructed to reduce its overall staffing. Efforts to meet current ceilings and further reductions to meet the President's goals will result in the loss of about 85 positions from the Shiprock service unit. This will only worsen the imbalance of needs and resources.

We would like to ask Congress to reinstate that waiver language for IHS. We hear from Washington that cuts in funding and staffing are only aimed at the future. I'm here to let you know that they are happening right now. We are told that cuts will not affect the health providers.

But the hiring freeze for the past five months resulted in losing dentists, doctors and nurses who wanted to come to work in Shiprock. Just this month, 13 employees received termination notices for budget reasons. These people provided direct services, including an OB nurse, two mental health counselors, two health educators, one women's health outreach worker, and other support personnel. This is only the first round of cuts, and it has already taken a significant negative impact on patient care and family services.

I serve on the interim education committee in the legislature. Yesterday we were talking about requiring in the State of New Mexico, in our curriculum, the Holocaust, the genocide that took place years ago. It makes one wonder how we're going to see, if this is going to be a fashion or some kind of a genocide that may result from lack of health care that we are witnessing today. Our population and our needs are growing, so we need more staff, not less. The IHS methodology calculates the need for 515 new positions. we need this.

The Chairperson from the Ute Tribe asked for some beds. This was 20 years ago, the design that was planned asked for 125 beds. So, 20 years ago, we were eligible for 125 beds. A few years ago, when the methodology kicked in, Shiprock was eligible for 165 beds for certain wards in our hospitals. The Inspector General said "Your hospitals are under-utilized, so you don't need those beds," and we were cut all the way down to 45 beds, and it went back up to 75.

Our population and our needs are growing, so we need more staff, not less. The resources to pay for the new staff is about $23 million per year. Even with this increase, Shiprock will spend about $990 per person, which is still below the overall IHS average of $1,132 and only one-fourth of the national health care spending of $3,760 per person.

We need relief from Federal employment ceilings, reduction plans and budget cuts. We want to follow through on plans to bring a wider range of services to our people in a more respectful manner with more reasonable waiting times. We want to maintain the programs for our community, the preventive health services. These programs realize savings in the long run.

Last but not least, we request, again, for language in the appropriation that the 515 new position and fund be specifically earmarked for Shiprock. We are afraid that IHS will use the new positions and funds to reduce its FTE and budget reduction and even allocate the new positions to other IHS programs. If reductions are to occur, it should happen at IHS headquarter level. We have too many chiefs and not enough Indians.

[Applause.]

Mr. Atcitty. Mr. Chairman, this concludes my statement. We will submit a more detailed briefing for your review and the record. I would be happy to answer any questions you may have.

We are planning our dedication on September 2, 1994, the Friday before Labor Day. Gentlemen, you are invited to come and celebrate with us on that day. We are also inviting you to take the time to tour the hospital construction and see what might be a white elephant. Thank you for your time.

[Applause.]

[Prepared statement of Mr. Atcitty appears in appendix.]

Senator McCain. Thank you very much, Mr. Atcitty, we appreciate your very compelling statement.

I would like to ask the rest of the witnesses to indulge me, I have to catch a plane in about on-half hour and I would appreciate it if you would attempt to keep your statements to about 5 minutes. I want to assure you that your complete statement will be made a part of the record, and that Senator Domenici and I will not only read all of your statements but share it with our fellow members of the committee. Thank you very much.

Ms. Hubbard-Pourier, please proceed, and welcome.

STATEMENT OF LYDIA HUBBARD-POURIER, EXECUTIVE DIRECTOR, NAVAJO DIVISION OF HEALTH

Ms. Hubbard-Pourier. Thank you very much, Senator McCain and Senator Domenici, Congressman Kyl. Thank you for the opportunity to briefly update you on the Hantavirus activity.

Before I proceed, I would like to thank publicly Senator Domenici on behalf of the Navajo people for your very prompt response to the funding for the Hantavirus activity back in May of last year, which started in May of last year. When Mr. Zah and myself came back to meet with the Congressional leaders on the Hantavirus outbreak in June of last year and in July, you were very prompt in assisting the Navajo Nation in requesting funding, not only for the Navajo Nation, but the Indian Health Service, the CDC and the National Institutes of Health, and certainly the New Mexico Health department.

You will be pleased to know that these funds are being put to good use in a number of areas. First of all, yesterday I was meeting with the health education and community health people, staff from the State of New Mexico, and our staff, Mr. Herman Shorty, the director of the community health programs, and our health education program for the Navajo Nation and the Indian Health Service Environmental Health Care are coordinating an additional campaign, since we are coming on the high-risk season again, that of spring and spring cleaning, and again the increase in the population of the deermouse.

First of all, one of the things that occurred last year in the outbreak is we all embarked on an extensive community education campaign in two areas, number one, getting information about symptomology and where to seek help and when to seek help to alleviate the problem among the Navajo people, who were extraordinarily affected by this mysterious illness.

The second part of the community education campaign then proceeded to get information to the community about cleanup, rodent abatement. The second part of that also then proceeded to a plan of rodent abatement activity. This rodent abatement task force included members of the Indian Health Service, the BIA and the Navajo Division of Health, and we were all going at this point.

We've done a preliminary assessment and find ourselves now to be experts in the United States on how to conduct campaigns on community education and also cleanup. Some of us are experts, including Mr. Herman Shorty, who is head our environmental health program in the Navajo Division of Health. We have learned how to trap rodents appropriately, how to help cleanup and how to do other kinds of things as well.

One of the things that came about, if you recall, the virus early on was thought to, there was a drug that was thought to possibly be effective in finding the Hantavirus, and the FDA and CDC worked together to allow for the extent of the use of this drug, the compassionate use of this drug on victims of the Hantavirus at that particular time.

However, under the rules and regulations of the FDA, this drug can no longer be utilized under compassionate use, and the National Institutes of Health and FDA and CDC are all pushing for an efficacy study on the procedures set out by the FDA. At some point in time, we are currently trying to implement that study, which will include the use of placebo for the Hantavirus.

These are ongoing activities. One of the things that was found during this time we were dealing with this experimental drug was that we found the Navajo Nation did have fairly good structures in looking at the research and the protection of subjects in the research. One of the outgrowth of the Hantavirus activity was that we are in the process of developing a research goal that will allow the Navajo Nation to assume control of this particular area of their own self-government.

The other area that we have worked very much with the Indian Health Service, and this is at the direction of the Navajo Health Services Committee, was to develop a medical surveillance program that would strongly reinforce the health departments when they were dealing with this and other diseases. And one of the things that has occurred just recently, we now are in the middle of a hepatitis outbreak and the communication links that were built between the various state health departments are kicking into place once again to help with that.

Of course, one of the major activities that went on was coordination of all of the inter-agency activity, between the national Federal agencies and the State Health Department as well, and the local Indian Health Service and the Navajo Nation. There was a lot of activity in health resources and a lot of agency people that worked together very, very well, and I think we're going to see the outcome of that to have continued networks of coordination in other areas, such as the hepatitis outbreak we just mentioned.

This all comes down to on area, that of a real need for a tribal government agency that deals with public health and community health. While Indian Health Service has specialized in the provision of medical services to Indian communities, we found that the Navajo Division of Health was very, very skillful in providing specific culturally sensitive community education activities.

The other area that we are very concerned about is of course the whole area of regulation and provision of public health services and community education. We feel that this is very, very critical. So when we're talking about public health, we're talking about public sanitation, environmental health, previous witnesses have discussed the importance of the 121 sanitation projects on the solid waste disposal.

All of these are very critical and probably do more to reduce the incidence of infectious diseases than anything else that anybody else would do, either by a nurse or a doctor. And you can tell I have a public health background, because I'm coming at it from that standpoint.

That is no to negate the critical need for personal medical services, but it also points out the real need for other public health services. Mr. Plummer indicated the foundation had been laid in Public Law 94–437 and in the 638 contracting self-determination act activities. All of these point to the need for a model which has been established through your guidance, through Congress' mandates, and legislative activity, that we do need to maintain the model that Indian Health Service has embarked upon utilizing, that of community-based public health models for provision of health and medical services to Native Americans.

In particular, we are very concerned because we feel this model has worked particularly well with the Navajo Nation Division of Health and its governmental agencies. And I would like to thank, on behalf of the Navajo Division of Health, you for coming and listening to our specific needs. We are concerned about the future of our 638 contracts for health services.

While we are now talking about budget cuts, specifically to Indian Health Service programs and the staffing of Indian Health Service, the Indian Health Service for the first 2 years has held its 638 grants and contracts back from having an effect on those cuts. However, as I understand from the leadership of the Indian Health Service, in the next 2 to 3 years, we are looking at cutbacks of tribal 638 grants and contracts as well, because the Indian Health Service will no longer be able to cut only its positions and budget.

So I thank you for that further impact that we foresee coming down the line to the Navajo Division of Health and its programs.

Senator McCain. Thank you very much.

STATEMENT OF NORMAN RATION, ACTING DIRECTOR, DEPARTMENT OF BEHAVIORAL HEALTH, NAVAJO DIVISION OF HEALTH

Mr. Ration. Senator McCain, Senator Domenici, Congressman Kyl, and President Zah thank you for allowing me to testify today.

As you know, Senator Domenici, we've worked on alcohol projects before together, and we know that there are many illnesses and accidents caused by alcohol and alcohol related activities. And we're here at the end of the day to talk to you about these same issues. As you know, it's a very grave problem on this reservation and other reservations.

To date, we have carried out a number of programs which have been successful, but are limited to outpatient kinds of programs and to residential types of treatment outside the reservation. One of the very important issues that we have here on Navajo is the need for having facilities here on Navajo, so we don't have to pay the exorbitant prices of going off-reservation to provide residential treatment for our members here.

The other issue is that most of the time when we send them off-reservation they are not culturally sensitive types of programs, and I wonder whether or not we are really able to accomplish what we send our people to these centers for. Several years ago, we worked together and got the Montonjorse Center in Gallup, and at that time we requested the assistance of Congress to provide funding for an adult treatment facility in Crown Point. And we have been given funds for that facility on a piecemeal basis, and 3 years later we're still trying to open the facility. And as we do some piecemeal construction, it gets vandalized, and again we fail to be able to open those facilities.

We're also known as a behavioral health program on Navajo and we have been doing pretty much alcohol kinds of activities. We are now embarking on mental health services that are very badly lacking on Navajo, even though there's a lot of coordination of activity between IHS and the Navajo Nation in trying to deliver services, we still find ourselves far short of delivering those services. So we are trying to ask some other programs to bring about those services on Navajo by working through state programs.

But to date we still have no day treatment program for the severely mentally ill, we have no long-term placement, we still have a lot of problems with fetal alcohol syndrome. We still have unavailability of inpatient psychiatric service for adults and children, and continue to have these problems.

The other area that I think we're very concerned with is that we send our people off to various kinds of treatment, but we don't have the education and prevention and intervention of our community members, so we try to work with the community members. We just started a new project for community mobilization and trying to work toward the multidisciplinary model that would involve a community member and family member in setting up a support system out in the community, which we think, as we work at it and have the necessary funding to carryout those kinds of activities, that we'll be able to return people back to their families with their necessary support system and be able to keep them from alcohol abuse and other substance abuse, and also to treat those that have a mental health problem with their abuse problems, which are all family-related kinds of health problems.

So we continue to move ahead in trying to put these different program together, but fall far short in terms of the availability of facilities, dollar resources and also staffing resources. But nonetheless, we continue to work toward that goal of hopefully achieving a more permanent kind of a program for all our community and family members through the Navajo Nation.

Thank you.

[Prepared statement of Mr. Ration appears in appendix.]

Senator McCain. Thank you very much, and thank you for all you're doing.

Do you have any questions?

Senator Domenici. How is the one in Gallup working?

Mr. RATION. The one in Gallup is working very well, as a matter of fact, they have a lot of clientele, and once they've sobered them up, then the issue becomes where do we send them, where do we refer them, and that's why there is a big need for a facility, because they don't have any place to refer them, because all the programs that we have subcontracted and we are working with utilize all the funds that we have available, and we feel that we could offer a better service if we had facilities on Navajo at less cost.

Senator MCCAIN. Thank you very much.

Our final three witnesses are Peggy Nakai, Roselyn Chapela, and Herman Shorty. Ms. Nakai, welcome and thank you.

STATEMENT OF PEGGY NAKAI, HEALTH PROGRAM MANAGER, OFFICE OF SPECIAL PROJECTS FOR THE NAVAJO DIVISION OF HEALTH

Ms. NAKAI. Thank you very much.

Good afternoon, Senator McCain and Senator Domenici, and Congressman Kyl and Mr. Zah. My name is Peggy Nakai, I am the Health Program Manager for the Office of Special Projects for the Navajo Division of Health. We appreciate this opportunity to present the Navajo Nation's comments and recommendations on the proposed fiscal year 1995 IHS budget reductions that directly impact the Navajo Area IHS health facilities and sanitation facilities. The Navajo Nation looks forward to working with you on these issues.

I will make this statement very brief, but I think you've heard it stated very well about Shiprock, Northern Navajo Medical Center, it's a nice hospital, where's the staff? I'd like to add that in addition to the $23 million that the Navajo Nation is requesting for the 515 additional staff, we are also asking for $2.9 million for activation expenses. We need these funds to be able to move into the new medical center. These funds will allow the staff to purchase necessary items like bedsheets, dishes, and those types of things.

On the Tohatchi Health Center, we are asking for $3.3 million, to also hire additional staff. This facility is 38,000 square feet and will serve the five communities in the area and will also accommodate for the overflow during the renovation of the Gallup Medical Center, which is scheduled to begin this summer.

For the Fort Defiance Hospital, we are requesting $37 million for the first-phase construction for this facility upon completion of the design phase in fiscal year 1995. IHS' 1995 budget does not include a request. So we have been asked to explore the possibility of this request. We are requesting approximately $5.1 million to conduct the site work and utilities work for the first phase.

The second phase will require $8.6 million to continue to complete the site work and utility and foundation work. The third phase requires approximately $14.2 million for the site work, utilities, foundation and superstructure. The final phase will require approximately $20 million to enclose the facility. These incremental processes will be forwarded in the next four fiscal years.

For the record, the health center is awaiting final approval of the proposed documents, the program requirements and program participation documents for the office headquarters. Recently an analysis was requested by the IHS regarding the feasibility of instituting the utilization of two facilities to serve the Navajo. The Navajo Nation supports this proposal, but requests more centrally located satellite facilities be considered. Further, expeditious review and approval is requested from IHS headquarters. We ask you for your support.

Another facility that we are asking for funds for is the Dilkon Health Center. The Navajo Nation is requesting a replacement facility for the Winslow Health Center. The Dilkon Committee has requested an appropriation in the amount of $21 million to construct a new health facility. The Winslow Health Center was condemned after the 1971 earthquake, and this facility is 64 years old, and just recently another analysis was done on the facility and that is a report by a consulting engineering firm from Albuquerque, New Mexico that states the facility should be demolished as soon as possible.

The IHS clinic building has been renovated over the years to the cost of over $1 million. The building is a health and safety hazard. There is inadequate space for patients waiting within the following areas: Examination rooms, waiting rooms, office rooms, x ray room, emergency room and isolation. The renovation program has caused other programs to be housed in large trailers, buildings and renovated buildings that are many years old, also. There is inadequate office space for staff. For example, physicians offices are in the main building, but their secretaries are situated in renovated patient restrooms within that building.

There is a high staff turnover. We are certain that it is attributable to the outdated facilities in which they are required to provide services. The health center is in a rural system, and causes clients to travel hundreds of miles, or health care needs go unmet. The Tuba City Hospital is hundreds of miles away, Gallup, NM is 130 miles away, the Chinle Hospital in Arizona is 140 miles away and also Phoenix is 360 miles away. These are one-way trips.

So we are asking your help in looking into this matter about the Winslow Hospital, and we are also asking for your support for the facility staff quarters for IHS staff that are badly needed also. This is a very essential requirement. As you know, we live in a very rural and isolated area out there on the reservation. Maintenance staff are required to be on a 24-hour call basis. And we just do not have adequate housing available for sale or rent anywhere on the reservation for these staff. So we are asking for your support in this area, too.

Also all over the world people dream of coming to America, but yet here on our own reservation, many people are enduring many hardships. One of the things that we have to endure, that many people have to endure every day, is hauling water so they can drink the water, so they can bathe, and water their livestock. Some of these people travel 50 and 60 miles round trip to haul water. We are asking your support to restore the $85 million that was cut from the IHS budget, $25 million of this money was being planned to be used to extend water lines to 500 families on the Navajo Reservation.

In conclusion, I would like to state that I have often heard the comment from the Indian Health Service that they are attempting to seek third-party payment for services, if only the tribe would pay. I would remind them that our forefathers have already paid a great price. As you travel throughout this great land, you will also remember that a great price has already been paid. These services are not free, they have been paid for by our ancestors prior to us seeking services.

Thank you very much.

[Prepared statement of Ms. Nakai appears in appendix.]

Senator McCAIN. Thank you very much.

Ms. Chapela.

STATEMENT OF ROSELYN CHAPELA, PROGRAM MANAGER, HIV/AIDS PROGRAM, NAVAJO DIVISION OF HEALTH

Ms. CHAPELA. Thank you very much.

Good afternoon, Senator McCain, Senator Domenici, and Congressman Kyl.

I am honored and grateful to present the status of the AIDS pandemic on the Navajo Nation to you this afternoon. As presented by John Hubbard, the Director of the Navajo Area IHS, AIDS, HIV/AIDS has affected the Navajo people. Although the Navajo people have a very, very strong and unique culture, AIDS does not respect culture.

Among the Navajo Nation, or among Native Americans and Alaska Natives, according to the IHS headquarters, as of September 1993, there were 731 report AIDS cases, 301 cases of which were from the southwestern region. As you recall, the Navajo Nation covers three States, and up to 301, as reported by Mr. Hubbard, 20 percent of the HIV cases are from the southwest region, which includes the Navajo Nation. As Mr. Hubbard indicated, 17 people have died from the Navajo people of AIDS, and 29 are living with HIV and 3 are living with AIDS.

This has adversely impacted the Navajo people, not only the immediate families, but the Navajo people are all feeling it through clanship or through blood. And more importantly and most alarming is that it's been recorded that the percentage of American Indians, women of child-bearing age with HIV is 4 to 8 times higher of that of the national average among women. That means, to give you a clear picture, according to the statistics on the Navajo Nation, 60 percent of the HIV or AIDS cases are women.

The other frightening situation is now the Navajo people, the Navajo children are having to be placed in foster homes. These children are HIV positive, and we have to begin dealing with families who don't know much about the care and the needs of special care and attention of these children. It links us with other programs such as social services, it links us with other programs such as the Department of Education, and then alcoholism and substance abuse.

Due to the long incubation period, HIV infection and AIDS diagnosis is about 10 years, so studies indicate that most of these women or in these cases, people have contracted AIDS or HIV when they were teens. So most of our focus in the Navajo Nation focuses on this youth population.

78-786 - 94 - 2

Until medical research finds a cure for AIDS, the Navajo Nation is very adamant about doing prevention education in the schools. We have a very unique program. We are using the Navajo foster grandparents to assist us in delivering prevention education messages to our children.

The other very important information that I would like to put into the record is the Navajo Nation Council understands the devastation and death of AIDS, and they understand the impact that these increased AIDS cases have among the Navajo people. As a result, in 1993, they appropriated funds to create an AIDS focus on the Navajo Nation, and the Navajo Nation has its first AIDS office this year.

And again, the Navajo Nation Council is also delivering the budget, and our budget has been severely cut. So we are looking up to Indian Health Service and possibly State agencies. And I am here today to urge the Senators and Congressman to support the Navajo Nation in implementing or mandating state operated schools to appropriate or incorporate AIDS education into their curriculum and also to mandate the Department of Education and Department of Health to support staff and other costs to implement these activities.

And most importantly, IHS cuts also impact the AIDS office. Because when it comes to basic medical care, the prevention programs are always the first ones to be cut. As indicated by Mr. Hubbard earlier, the CDC is cutting their prevention and education programs. So the way we see it is that if prevention and education funding could be restored, it will eventually in the long run save basic medical care and also save Navajo-wide, including the Navajo people.

Thank you.

Senator McCain. Thank you.

Mr. Shorty, welcome.

STATEMENT OF HERMAN SHORTY, PROGRAM COORDINATOR, OFFICE OF ENVIRONMENTAL HEALTH, NAVAJO DIVISION OF HEALTH

Mr. Shorty. Thank you, and welcome, Mr. Chairman, Senator Domenici and Congressman Kyl, and President Zah.

I appreciate the opportunity to come before you and take our testimony as well and speak on behalf of the Navajo Nation.

The environmental health problems are similar to those communities that you all are from. The objective and goals of the Division of Health and my mission for the Office of Environmental Health is to effectively reduce morbidity and mortality rates that are recorded, and those that may be reported in the future.

Environmental health problems and concerns encompass injuries, water and sewer services, environmental diseases, and solid waste. In a single word, this means prevention. As what was experienced and what will be experienced in FTE cuts will be in the area of prevention as well, because it is here that we're looking at prevention before they go to the medical facilities for services.

Regarding injuries on Navajo Nation, the injury rate is high. The leading cause of death among Navajos is injuries. It is at a rate of

4½ times that of the national average, a rate twice as high as the next leading cause, which is heart disease. Injury deaths are seen from motor vehicle crashes predominantly.

Just to give you an overall picture or snapshot of what the Navajo Nation is faced with, reports for 1993: In accidents alone with injuries recorded was 68; with deaths, 49; homicide, 15; aggravated assaults, 314; assaults and batteries, 2,384; sex offenses, 364; offenses family and child, 576; suicide and attempts alone for the first quarter of 1994 have been 10, 3 suicides and 7 attempts. What's not reflected here is the cost associated with prevention, response and care associated with injuries in each one of those categories.

In the areas of environmental diseases, for the Navajo Nation, environmental related disease is a serious and real concern. With the recent outbreak of Hantavirus, it has become evident that cultural values and the traditional methods of health in preventing diseases must never be lost. In addition to that, we appreciate the support that we have received from Congress and the response that was given as far as the outbreak was concerned. It has been my understanding that the response was the magnitude of 10 man years that was focused in on this response.

Additional environmental concerns for the Navajo Nation is hepatitis A, shigella, salmonella, rabies, plague, and now Hantavirus. Congressional support in the form of adequate funding shall provide good, sound environmental health programs and effective practices. Provisions of how the water, waste disposal from the sanitation procedures, food sanitation and marketing, environmental health conditions of the schools, restaurants, hospitals, nursing homes, and water systems, surveillance of those carrying plague and Hantavirus and rabies all contribute to reducing the rates of environmentally related diseases. The proposal of FTE reduction and cuts certainly affects these areas, gentlemen.

Solid waste is also another concern. The Navajo Nation is not immune to the trails of visible blight that leaves few corners of our country unspotted with refuse on land. Litter along the roadside, abandoned vehicles, thousands of open dumps scar our land. As you well know, residential, commercial, institutional, and industrial solid waste are a serious threat to health and the environment. They are the most offensive and the most dangerous to health.

An overriding concern is the disposal of discarded hazardous waste—those, by virtue of their composition and longevity are harmful, toxic or lethal.

On the Navajo Nation, there are approximately 350 dumpsites that would qualify for the open dump list identified by authorities for abatement. Of these numbers, 150 to 200 may be the subject of proper closure procedures. The remainder would require corrective measures to upgrade them to meet the required standards to remain operative.

Not reflected here, however, are the thousands of small family camp sites or community dumps, and illegal dumping areas. The priority, from my understanding from Navajo EPA, is that the priority on the Navajo Nation is to focus in on the development of three approved sanitary landfill sites. The initial proposed approximate costs for design and development is about $3 million per site, for a total of $10 million for the proposed process.

That concludes my testimony before this distinguished panel. Thank you.

Senator McCAIN. Thank you very much.

Senator DOMENICI. I have no questions, Mr. Chairman, but I do want to extend to you my gratitude for your coming to New Mexico to conduct this hearing, and bringing Representative Kyl with you. I want to thank Peterson Zah, President of the Navajo Nation, for inviting us here, and all of you for helping us with your testimony. We work together very well, Senator McCain and I, and we have a lot of other supporters in the United States Senate, and we're going to try our best, with your help, to make some inroads in these areas that you have shared with us today which you think are very important to your people, and we join with you in that concern.

Thank you very much, and thank you, Senator McCain.

Senator McCAIN. Thank you very much for your kind hospitality, as always. Senator Domenici, I also want to thank the people here at Shiprock High School for allowing us to use their facility, and I want to thank all of our witnesses, including so many dedicated servants, public servants, for serving our Nation and the Navajo Nation with such honor and distinction, and I want to thank you and assure you that we've all learned a great deal, and we'll go back with some renewed vigor in attempting to do the Lord's work in the city of Satan.

Thank you very much, this hearing is adjourned.

[Whereupon, at 5 p.m., the committee was adjourned, to reconvene at the call of the Chair.]

APPENDIX

Additional Material Submitted for the Record

Prepared Statement of Hon. Jon Kyl, U.S. Representative from Arizona

Mr. Chairman, I appreciate the chance to join you and other members of the Senate Committee on Indian Affairs here today to examine the funding needs of the Indian Health Service (IHS).

Mr. Chairman, you will. recall that I represented a large portion of the Navajo Nation before House District lines were redrawn in 1992. Although my District has changed, my concern about issues affecting the Navajo people has not—particularly with respect to health care.

And that is what brings me here today to express my deep disappointment with the budget President Clinton has proposed for the IHS, and the impact it is sure to have on health care delivery for the Navajo people.

The President's FY 95 budget request, for example, includes enough funding to hire only about one-third of the staff necessary to fully staff and utilize the new Shiprock hospital. It makes little sense to have invested so much in the construction of this facility, only to have much of it idled by staff cuts now.

I would point out that this is not an area that is overserved. Waiting lists for care at IHS facilities are long, and people who are sick or injured often have to be transported on dirt roads up to a hundred miles to receive care. Life expectancy among Navajos is well under the U.S. average, and infant deaths far exceed those of the overall U.S. population. This is an area of significant need.

As the President of the Navajo Nation, Peterson Zah, wrote in a recent letter to me, "There is simply no logic in nor humanity in reducing health care services to those who so desperately need them."

We need to set better priorities in the Congress. A fifth of the Health and Human Services Department's staff cuts should not be borne by the IHS alone as is proposed for 1995. Health care should not be taken away from the very population that needs it most.

Cutting government spending does not have to mean across-the-board cuts or devastating cuts in the most important programs. It does mean rethinking priorities, eliminating the wasteful, obsolete or unnecessary programs, and putting off the luxuries for another day.

Mr. Chairman, I want to submit for the record a copy of President Zah's letter, as well as letters from Genevieve Jackson and other tribal leaders in Arizona about the proposed budget cuts. I also look forward to working with you and my colleagues in the House for a budget that better reflects the needs of this community.

Thank you.

STATEMENT OF THE NAVAJO NATION
Before the
SENATE COMMITTEE ON INDIAN AFFAIRS
On The
HEALTH CONCERNS & NEEDS OF THE NAVAJO NATION

Presented by
NAVAJO NATION PRESIDENT PETERSON ZAH

April 8,1994

SHIPROCK, NEW MEXICO

INTRODUCTION

Good Afternoon. Senator Pete V. Domenici, Senator John McCain and Congressman Jon Kyl. On behalf of the Navajo people and as President of the Navajo Nation, I present our concerns on fundamental and basic health care needs of the Navajos. I would especially like to thank Senators Domenici and McCain for their firm commitment of attempting to raise the health status of American Indians, particularly of the Navajo people. It is a monumental occasion to hold this field hearing here in Shiprock, New Mexico, the site of the newly constructed Northern Navajo Medical Center.

As you are well aware, the Navajo Nation is primarily served by the Indian Health Service (IHS) which is experiencing deep budget cuts and staff reductions in FY 1994 and 1995. Should the proposed FY 1995 IHS budget be implemented the reduction will adversely affect the delivery of primary health care services by not providing additional staffing for the new Shiprock hospital, funding for facilities construction, funding for important health programs, and funding for adequate medical staff.

Recently, the Navajos have begun to fully utilize the IHS. Historically, many Navajo were hesitant to seek health care services from IHS but the IHS reoriented its medical services to be sensitive to the Navajo culture. It has managed to communicate with traditional and illiterate Navajos that health care services are available at the IHS for all Navajo people. Consequently, the Navajo Area IHS is experiencing a substantially increase in patient load. The ill-proportioned primary care providers to Navajo patients continues to grow without relief to the depleted IHS budget or its primary care providers.

According to IHS data, American Indians are susceptible to a wide variety of illnesses and accidents. In some cases these higher death rates are quite substantial which include alcoholism, diabetes, tuberculosis and accidents. The health needs of the Navajo are particularly acute and are compounded by the low income level of our population. Fifty-three (53) percent of tribal members live in households with income level below the poverty level. Seventy-five (75) percent of Navajo homes have no phone service therefore many Navajo families do not have direct cr immediate health care access.

I do not understand how the Administration is advocating for health care reform and universal health care coverage for each citizen of this Country, yet, the Administration proposed FY 1995 IHS budget cuts and FTE reductions which contradicts the Administration's proposed Health Security Act (H.R. 3600).

I met with the Office of Management and Budget, the Department of Health and Human Services (HHS) and the IHS, they all cited the following four reasons to cut the IHS budget and reduce FTEs: (1) fat and fraud in IHS is not uniform throughout IHS. Historically, IHS has been understaffed especially in the Navajo Area IHS which results in 60 percent of the Navajo population to be underserved. The underserved Navajo and other Indian population should be carefully studied, then maybe HHS can determine where regional cuts should be made. HHS cuts should not be made across the board. (2) "638" compacting and contracting can save dollars and create employment opportunities for Indians. The practice of "638" compacting and contracting to create savings is a fallacy. If the IHS is already underfunded and underserved, how can Indian tribes effectively operate "638" compacting and contracting services with limited funds and past evidence of short falls. Moreover, the process of "638" compacting and contracting takes two to three years to complete, whereas IHS budget cuts and FTE reductions are being implemented now. (3) FTE cuts are only being made at the mid-level management of IHS. The mid-level management at IHS are in fact the physicians at grade level GS 14 and 15, clinicians and supervisors. These individuals provide direct health care services to Navajos. Further, the FTE reductions affect the part-time employees and other support staff which are mostly Navajos. Since IHS is one of the major employers on the Navajo reservation, these FTE reductions would increase unemployment on the Navajo Nation. (4) IHS can contract non-essential health services such as housekeeping, lab work, and food services. Contracting non-essential health services off the Navajo Nation creates Navajo unemployment in IHS and increases contracting expenses. For example, ninety-eight (98) percent of the Navajo Area IHS employees are Navajo and the FTE reductions have already and will eliminate jobs for Navajos. It seems that contracting off the reservation would be more expensive for IHS overall.

As a result of my meeting with HHS, Secretary Donna Shalala sent a letter on March 23, 1994 to OMB Director Leon Panetta requesting reconsideration of a FTE reduction waiver for Indian Health Service (IHS) in FY 1994 and FY 1995. Secretary Shalala emphasized that Congress viewed the FTE reductions for IHS in FY 1994 and FY 1995 unfavorably. She also indicated that the FTE reductions are inconsistent with the Health Care Reform initiatives outlined by President Clinton.

I am particularly pleased with Senator Domenici's letter dated March 9, 1994 to President Clinton, expressing concerns on the impact of the proposed federal staffing reductions and the elimination of additional staffing for those IHS health facilities which are scheduled to open this year. Senator Domenici stressed the inflated IHS projection that private collections from Medicare and Medicaid and other private insurance will make up substantial amounts of funding for the necessary FTEs. In President Clinton's response, it was very apparent that the Administration is totally unaware of the harsh impact the FTE reduction will have on the Navajo Area IHS, especially with the impact of inadequate staffing at the Shiprock hospital. I am disturbed that the Administration promises us enhanced health care services through Health Care Reform, yet the Administration drastically cuts the IHS budget. Ultimately, the Navajo people are the ones who will suffer.

Thank you, Senator McCain, for expressing the Navajo Nation's concerns on the adverse impacts of the FTE reductions and referencing my letter to you before the Senate Committee on Indian Affairs hearing on March 3, 1994. I appreciate your support for the Shiprock hospital and the need for additional staffing.

RECOMMENDATIONS

The Navajo Nation requests Congress' assistance to waive the FTE reduction in IHS and to restore full funding for IHS. We request an increase in the IHS budget to further upgrade the current health care system which has been funded at only 68 percent of the total health care need.

In addition, the Navajo Nation specifically requests Congress to include further funding for an additional 515 FTEs and activation cost for the Northern Navajo Medical Center located in Shiprock, New Mexico.

The Navajo Nation recommends that language be included in the appropriations legislation that would prevent any further budget cuts and staff reductions in IHS.

CONCLUSION

We believe that health care reform must ensure that every citizen including American Indians are provided quality health care. The third panel of Navajo health professional will expand on these health concerns of the Navajo Nation.

We thank Senators Domenici and McCain and Congressman Kyl for hearing our concerns on health care. We also appreciate Chairman Daniel Inouye and the Senate Committee on Indian Affairs for their support on ensuring Indians are fairly included in health care reform.

Genevieve Jackson

NAVAJO NATION TESTIMONY ON CHILD ABUSE ISSUES

before

Senators John McCain and Pete V. Domenici

and

Congressman Jon Kyl
April 18, 1994

The Navajo Nation testimony on child abuse issues will provide a briefing on the current foundation for continuing the development and implementation of the Navajo Child Abuse and Neglect Five Year Plan; a summary of achievements and year-end summaries of the Navajo Child Sexual Abuse Project (NCSAP); and recommendations for improvements and development of the NCSAP and other child abuse related programs.

HISTORICAL INFORMATION

Community Advocacy Community (CAC)

In August 1990, a multi-agency Navajo Nation Ad Hoc Committee on child sexual abuse was organized to seek ways for improving the response of existing organizations to child sexual abuse and neglect cases on the Navajo Nation. In August 1992, the Navajo Nation Child Protection Team merged with the CAC. The CAC has dual roles of (1) being an oversight body for the local child protection teams on the Navajo Nation; and (2) serving as an advisory and advocacy body for the NCSAP. The CAC is comprised of multi-disciplinary professionals which coordinate preventive and protective services for Navajo child abuse victims and their families on the Navajo Nation. CAC seeks continual acknowledgement, support and cooperation from all entities involved in the NCSAP.

Comprehensive Five Year Plan

In October 1990, Congress earmarked funding in the FY'91 Interior Appropriations for the NCSAP. In the Spring of 1990, the Ad Hoc Committee completed the development of a comprehensive five year plan to enable the Navajo Nation and other organizations to make incremental steps (year-by-year) in addressing child abuse issues, starting in 1991 and ending in 1996. The Ad Hoc Committee identified NCSAP demonstration sites at Tuba City and Fort Defiance, Arizona and Shiprock, New Mexico to begin in the fall of 1990. However, due to funding misappropriation at the area level, NCSAP was not able to provide services until September of 1991 (FY'92).

At the beginning of FY'92, the three NCSAPs were unsuccessful in hiring qualified specialist for the three treatment teams. Late in FY'92, Tuba City NCSAP was finally able to hire its treatment team. At the end of FY'92, Fort Defiance NCSAP and Shiprock NCSAP hired treatment staff members.

Hence, FY'93 was the first full year of operation for the three treatment teams. The Navajo Nation was also committed to combating child abuse by appropriating general funds to establish NCSAPs in Crownpoint, New Mexico and Chinle, Arizona.

Multi-Disciplinary Approach to Treatment

The symptoms and causes of child sexual abuse and neglect are multi-faceted; hence treatment and prevention must be comprehensive and multi-disciplinary. The NCSAP provides treatment services that are holistic and customized to the needs of Navajo clientele. Victims of severe cases of child sexual abuse and neglect require long term care and services.

The NCSAP implements a multi-disciplinary response to child sexual abuse and neglect cases which involves a variety of human services professionals such as social workers, Navajo traditional counselors, mental health specialists, prosecutors, criminal investigators, attorneys, law enforcement officials, and the FBI.

ACHIEVEMENTS SINCE BEGINNING OF NCSAP

Prevention

The NCSAP aims to prevent child abuse incidences by educating the at-risk and general population of the Navajo Nation of child abuse issues. NCSAP has developed educational initiatives such as community-based responses to prevention and how and when to report incidences of child sexual abuse and neglect.

Treatment Services

NCSAP utilizes a multi-disciplinary and eclectic approach to therapy. Treatment teams integrate both Western and Navajo traditional approaches to individual, family and group therapy.

In order to further develop NCSAP, NCSAP would like to continue being involved in Congressional legislation to ensure support of our NCSAP efforts, developing protocols for child protection teams, and processing procedures for networking, and coordinating multi-disciplinary services.

Summary of NCSAP Activities from FY'92 to FY'94

FY'92 - First Year of NCSAP (9/91 to 9/92):

The treatment team at each of the five NCSAP received specialized training in various topics such as individual, family and group therapy for child sexual abuse and neglect victims. The treatment teams also received orientation and training in developing and administrating Child Protection Team (CPT) and Multi-Disciplinary Team (MDT) protocol and therapy protocols. Finally, the treatment teams learned the techniques of integrity of evidence for the prosecution of perpetrators.

The treatment teams at Tuba City and Fort Defiance, Arizona and Shiprock, New Mexico did not provide comprehensive treatment services for child sexual abuse victims until the end of FY'92. NCSAP provided Western and Navajo traditional therapy for individual's, families and groups. The three treatment teams served the following number of clientele: 99 primary victims, 43 secondary clientele (family members of victim) and 199 family members. The treatment teams also logged approximately 1,499 hours of contact time with their clientele for the first year.

The Tuba City treatment team was fortunate to begin their treatment services for child sexual abuse and neglect victims five months before either of the treatment teams at Fort Defiance, Arizona and Shiprock, New Mexico. During their first year, the Tuba City treatment team provided the following treatment services: 13 Navajo therapeutic ceremonies, 8 Navajo traditional therapeutic diagnostics and 12 Native American therapeutic services.

The Navajo Nation Office of the Prosecutors developed a draft protocol to coordinate a multi-disciplinary response to child sexual abuse and neglect on the Navajo Nation.

The Navajo Nation began initiatives to strengthen the Navajo Nation Children Code and Navajo Criminal Code to adequately protect child sexual abuse and neglect victims.

FY'93 - Second Year of NCSAP (9/92 to 9/93):

FY'93 was the first full year of operation for the three NCSAP at Tuba City and Fort Defiance, Arizona and Shiprock, New Mexico.

NCSAP conducted prevention seminars at 23 Navajo chapters, 13 boarding and public schools on the Navajo Nation. NCSAP conducted 4 radio broadcasts. NCSAP also distributed educational information on child sexual abuse issues at tribal fairs and various public functions. Over 700 Navajo families were contacted through prevention educational initiatives.

Aside from typical training on various techniques of clinical therapy the treatment teams took advantage of a seminar training which further enhanced the specialized therapy skills of the therapists including treatment services for offenders.

The three treatment teams logged about 2,235 hours and served 157 primary victims, 41 secondary clientele and about 257 family members. Although the nominal figure for contact time increased from the previous year, the percentage of contact time with clients decreased by over 10 per cent. NCSAP believes that the nominal decrease in therapy contact hours is related to the development of protocols, improvement of statistical reporting and establishment of local CPTs and MDTs during the second year of the project.

The Health and Social Services Committee of the Navajo Nation (oversight committee for the Navajo Division of Social Services) developed and adapted the Navajo Nation Child Protection protocol.

The Navajo Tribal Council adopted a Domestic Violence Prevention Act in August, 1993.

FY'94 - Year Three (9/93 to 9/94, Current Year)

From January, 1994, to March 30, 1994 prevention specialists visited 8 Navajo chapters, coordinated 2 information booths, conducted 2 radio announcements, distributed over 600 information packets and brochures on child abuse and neglect prevention. Over 1,000 Navajo children, families and citizens were informed of child abuse issues.

Training for therapist will continue. NCSAP would like other members of CPTs and MDTs to have access to training during this year.

Tuba City, Fort Defiance and Shiprock treatment teams logged about 1338 hours of contact time for 286 primary clientele and 194 secondary clientele during the first quarter of FY 94. The Crownpoint and Chinle treatment teams were not fully operational during the first quarter.

Currently, NCSAP is in the process of updating yearly Memorandum Of Agreements to reflect the changes in agency directors of BIA, IHS, and BIA-OIEP.

RECOMMENDATIONS TO IMPROVE AND DEVELOP NCSAP

The Navajo Nation provides the following recommendations:

(1) The Navajo Nation recommends that federal funds to NCSAP and other child abuse related programs are "re-occurring" so that current initiatives within the NCSAP are developed and improved. The Navajo Nation would like to continue providing and improving intervention, treatment and prevention services to Navajo child abuse victims and their families in a timely and efficient manner.

(2) In order to avoid further funding problems of NCSAP monies at the agency level, the Navajo Nation recommends that the NCSAP at the Central Office in Window Rock, Arizona receive federal appropriations directly from the federal source instead of through the current process of receiving federal funding from the BIA and IHS local agencies. The NCSAP did not really develop until the third year of funding because of miscommunication and problems with the federal agencies disbursing the funding to NCSAP in the first and second year.

(3) The Navajo Nation urges Congress and the Administration to provide full funding for P.L. 101-630, the Indian Child Protection and Family Violence Act. We are disappointed that the Administration did not request any funding for P.L. 101-630 in the FY'95 Budget and never has appropriated any funding for the Act since the enactment of P.L. 101-630.

(4) The Navajo Nation request Congress and the administration to require the CPTs of BIA Boarding School to participate and be a part of the local community CPTs and MDTs for comprehensive services for child abuse victims across the Navajo Nation.

The Navajo Nation appreciates and thanks Senators McCain and Domenici and Congressman Kyl for their support of Indian child abuse programs and services.

APRIL 8, 1994
FIELD HEARING - SHIPROCK, NM
PROPOSED HEALTH SECURITY ACT

IMPACT OF IHS BUDGET CUTS

PRESENTED BY:
JUDY KNIGHT-FRANK
CHAIRMAN, UTE MOUNTAIN UTE TRIBE
TOWAOC, COLORADO

THE SHIPROCK INDIAN HOSPITAL IS ONLY AVAILABLE TO THE UTE MOUNTAIN UTE TRIBE FOR INPATIENT CARE 25% OF THE TIME.

THIS RESULTED IN OUR CONTRACT HEALTH SERVICE EXPENDING APPROXIMATELY $279,000 MORE TO PRIVATE SECTOR HOSPITALS IN FY '93.

WE ANTICIPATED AND PLANNED THAT THE NEW HOSPITAL AT SHIPROCK WOULD CORRECT THIS INACCESSIBILITY AND DEFICIENCY BUT... THE PROPOSED FTE REDUCTIONS WILL NEGATE ANY POSITIVE PROGRESS WITHIN THE IHS FOR SERVICE TO ITS CLIENTS.

HOW CAN A BRAND NEW HOSPITAL JUST COMING ON LINE FUNCTION EFFECTIVELY AND EFFICIENTLY WITH THE PROPOSED CUTS?

THIS HOSPITAL IS SCHEDULED TO SERVE TRIBAL POPULATIONS THAT ARE IN A GROWTH MODE. THE TWO MAJOR POPULATIONS OF THE AREA BEING THE NAVAJO AND UTE POPULATIONS.

AS CHAIRMAN OF THE UTE MOUNTAIN UTE TRIBE, I WANT TO BRING TO YOUR ATTENTION THE SERVICE PROVIDED FROM OUR SMALL CLINIC IN TOWAOC WHICH SHOULD SERVICE 1900

PEOPLE, BUT SERVES 8500 CASES MOSTLY FROM OTHER INDIAN NATIONS.

HOW CAN WE WITH SUCH A SMALL STAFF WORK UNDER THE IMPENDING FTE PROPOSED CUTS, WHEN THE NEAREST HOSPITAL ALSO FACES FTE CUTS AND WE ARE ONLY ALLOWED 25% INPATIENT CARE ??

THE SHIPROCK HOSPITAL SHOULD PROVIDE A SPECIFIC NUMBER OF BEDS AS THIS WOULD ASSURE ACCESSIBILITY AND ALLEVIATE THE ROADBLOCKS OUR PEOPLE AND OUR IHS PERSONNEL EXPERIENCE. THE UTE MOUNTAIN UTE TRIBE WOULD BE GLAD TO FURNISH PATIENT INFORMATION TO MAKE THIS BED ALLOCATION

THE UTE MOUNTAIN UTE TRIBE IS THE LARGER RESIDENT TRIBE OF THE STATE OF COLORADO AND OUR SMALL UNDERSIZED CLINIC AND UNDER ALLOCATED FTE'S FOR OUR SIZE TRIBE ARE HANDLING AN EXTREMELY LARGE CASE LOAD.

IN FY' 92 OUTSIDE CARE COSTS WERE $241,000, FY '93 COSTS WERE $279,000, FY '94 JUST IN 6 MONTHS COSTS ARE OVER $250,000.

IF THE SHIPROCK HOSPITAL WOULD BE PROPERLY STAFFED AND SERVICES WERE AVAILABLE TO THE UTE TRIBE, THESE COSTS WOULD NOT HAVE OCCURRED.

WHERE IS THE LOGIC OF BUILDING A NEW HOSPITAL, NOT BEING ABLE TO STAFF IT AND NOT PROVIDING SERVICE FOR THE PEOPLE IT IS SUPPOSED TO SERVE? IF SHIPROCK INDIAN HOSPITAL BEDS WERE ACCESSIBLE TO THE UTE MOUNTAIN UTE PATIENTS, MOST OF THESE CHS DOLLARS COULD BE SAVED AND UTILIZED FOR SERVICES NOT AVAILABLE THROUGH THE IHS SYSTEM. WE ARE TOLD INACCESSIBILITY FOR OUR PEOPLE TO SHIPROCK IS THE RESULT OF NO BEDS AND PERSONNEL BEING 'RELUCTANT' TO ACCEPT NON NAVAJO PATIENTS. WHAT IF OUR SMALL CLINIC HAD THESE QUALMS ? WHAT IF OUR

SMALL CLINIC GAVE THESE OTHER NATIVE AMERICANS PATIENTS THE 'RUN AROUND' SIMILAR TO THE PROBLEMS WE FACE WHEN TRYING TO TRANSFER A PATIENT TO SHIPROCK. THIS IS JUST ONE MORE EXAMPLE AS TO WHY THE COSTS OF CHS DOLLARS ARE SO HIGH. THE SHIPROCK HOSPITAL **MUST** SERVICE THE NATIVE AMERICAN PEOPLE OF OUR AREA AND **MUST** SERVICE THEM WELL TO PREVENT THE OUTSIDE CHS COSTS TO CONTINUE TO RISE AND **MUST** NOT TAKE ANY FUNDING CUTS.

I KNOW OUR TREATIES CALL FOR HEALTH SERVICE TO BE PROVIDED TO THE TRIBES AND WITH THE SERVICE WE NOW RECEIVE, WE, THE UTE MOUNTAIN UTE TRIBE HAVE LOOKED FOR OUTSIDE HEALTH INSURANCE FOR ITS WORKING TRIBAL MEMBERS. THE $280.00 MONTHLY FAMILY PLAN COST IS MORE THAN MOST OF OUR EMPLOYEES CAN AFFORD ON HOURLY WAGES. THE TRIBE AFTER SEEKING CARE FOR ITS MEMBERS THEN IS INFORMED THAT THE IHS IS NOT CONSIDERED A PRIME CARE PROVIDER.

WHY DID WE HAVE TO GO TO SUCH LENGTHS WHEN THE TREATIES CALL FOR THE US GOVERNMENT TO PROVIDE THIS SERVICE ?

THANK YOU FOR GIVING ME THE OPPORTUNITY TO TESTIFY BEFORE THIS HEARING TODAY, WE WILL BE SUBMITTING FURTHER DOCUMENTATION FOR THE RECORD.

DEPARTMENT OF HEALTH & HUMAN SERVICES

Public Health Service

Indian Health Service
Indian Health Clinic
Towaoc, Colorado 81334

MEMORANDUM

Date: February 7, 1994

From: Health Center Director, Towaoc Health Center

Subject: Navajo Usage of Towaoc Health Center

The Towaoc Health Center computer data base has 7555 patients entered. Of those, 4891 (65%) are Navajo. The geographic distribution is incredible.

1. We have 1201 Navajo patients living in Utah: Aneth (379), Blanding (181), Bluff (63), Montezuma Creek (560), Monticello (13) and Red Mesa (5). Note Montezuma Creek has a five day a week Health Center and all of the listed communities are closer to Montezuma Creek than to the Towaoc Health Center. Aneth, Montezuma Creek and Red Mesa are on the Navajo Reservation.

2. We have 809 Navajo patients living in the Shiprock area: Farmington (51), Fruitland (28), Hogback (12), Kirtland (20), Waterflow (21) and Shiprock (677). Shiprock Indian Hospital is located on the Navajo Reservation and is one of the five largest Indian Health Service Hospitals in operation. These patients actually must drive by that facility to get to ours.

3. Teec Nos Pos has a five day a week IHS Health Center yet we have 180 Navajo patients from there.

4. Cortez is in Shiprock's "Health Care Delivery Area" yet we have 1522 Navajo patients living there who have accessed the Towaoc Health Center. WE HAVE Literally MORE NAVAJO PATIENTS IN CORTEZ THAN WE HAVE UTE patients in TOWAOC (1522 vs 1385).

5. Of interest, are the Navajo patients who live in communities with large IHS facilities (besides those already mentioned) yet have driven to Towaoc to use this Health Center:

   Albuquerque - 12
   Chinle - 21
   Crownpoint - 10
   Kayenta - 19
   Tuba City - 05
   Gallup - 05

The above indicates the tremendous impact on our direct care services but the Navajo population has also impacted our Contract Health Service budget. By moving onto the Ute Mountain Ute Reservation the Navajo patients become eligible for our already over burdened CHS monies. There are presently 285 Navajo living in Towaoc and 56 Navajo living in White Mesa. The Navajo represent 16% of the total White Mesa population and access care through our agreement with the Blanding Medical Center and we are forced by CHS regulation to pay.

Our Contract Health Service Delivery Area overlaps the Shiprock Contract Health Service Area and the regulations have hurt us and helped them.

The reasons for using our facility are varied but usually involve a shorter waiting time as a non-appointment at our facility versus a longer waiting time with an appointment at the Navajo Area facility. Theoretically, our patients can access care at the Navajo facilities but they are virtually inaccessible. This is especially true on the inpatient side. Nine out of ten times our patients are turned down for inpatient care with the excuse "no beds are available". This again places a hugh burden on our CHS budget.

Ronnie D. Thomas, HCD

Ronnie D. Thomas, HCD
Towaoc, CO

TESTIMONY OF STATE REP. THOMAS E. ATCITTY

CHAIRMAN,
SHIPROCK HOSPITAL STEERING COMMITTEE
SHIPROCK, NEW MEXICO

GOOD AFTERNOON, MR. CHAIRMAN, SENATOR DOMENICI, CONGRESSMAN KYL, PRESIDENT ZAH, VICE PRESIDENT PLUMMER AND PANEL MEMBERS. THANK YOU FOR OFFERING THE SHIPROCK HOSPITAL STEERING COMMITTEE THIS OPPORTUNITY TO TESTIFY ON THE NEED FOR ADDITIONAL STAFFING FOR THE NEW SHIPROCK HOSPITAL AND THE IMPACT OF THE FTE REDUCTION. HONORABLE CONGRESSMEN, I DO NOT NEED TO EDUCATE YOU ON THE IMPORTANCE OF QUALITY HEALTH CARE SERVICES FOR THE NAVAJO PEOPLE. YOU ACKNOWLEDGED OUR NEED FOR A NEW HOSPITAL IN SHIPROCK BY APPROPRIATING $53 MILLION FOR THE PLANNING/DESIGN AND CONSTRUCTION OF A REPLACEMENT FACILITY IN FY '87, '92 AND '93. UNFORTUNATELY, THE PRESIDENT'S FY '95 BUDGET DOES NOT CONTAIN ANY MONIES TO FULLY STAFF AND OPERATE THE NEW NORTHERN NAVAJO MEDICAL CENTER.

IN SHIPROCK, WE HAVE 4 TIMES AS MANY PATIENTS PER DOCTOR AS THE NATIONAL RATIO. THE 515 NEW POSITIONS WILL IMPROVE THE RATIO AND MAKE IT EASIER FOR OUR PEOPLE TO SEE THE SAME DOCTOR AND RECEIVE SUFFICIENT TIME FOR A THOROUGH EXAMINATION. BUT ANY INCREASE IN THE NUMBER OF PROVIDERS REQUIRES AN ADDITIONAL INCREASE IN SUPPORT STAFF, SUCH AS NURSING, LAB, X-RAY AND MEDICAL RECORDS. WITHOUT ANY NEW NURSES AND SUPPORT STAFF, WE CAN FORGET ABOUT OUR PLANS FOR NEW SPECIALTY SERVICES, SPECIALIZED SURGERY SUCH AS OPHTHALMOLOGY, UROLOGY AND ENT.

IF WE CANNOT INCREASE OUR STAFF, WHO WILL CLEAN OUR BEAUTIFUL NEW HOSPITAL? WILL PATIENTS HAVE TO MOP THEIR OWN ROOMS AND CHANGE LIGHTBULBS? WHO WILL OPERATE THE NEW AND MUCH NEEDED MEDICAL EQUIPMENT, LIKE THE CT SCANNER? IF OUR X-RAY TECHNICIANS ARE ASSISTING WITH CT SCANS, ROUTINE DIAGNOSTIC X-RAY AND ULTRASOUND

TESTS WILL HAVE TO BE DEFERRED. OR, DO WE NOT USE THE SCANNER AND REFER PATIENTS TO OUTSIDE HOSPITALS WHICH IS VERY EXPENSIVE?

HOW WILL WE KEEP UP WITH OUR INCREASING MEDICAL NEEDS SUCH AS DIABETES, HIGH BLOOD PRESSURE, HEART DISEASE, AND THE GROWING NEEDS OF OUR FAMILIES AND COMMUNITIES?

DECISIONS THAT ONLY FOCUS ON DIRECT MEDICAL CARE ARE A THREAT TO OUR COMMUNITY HEALTH PROGRAMS. WE HAVE A COMMITMENT TO ALL THE PEOPLE WITHIN THE COMMUNITY - REACHING OUT WITH PUBLIC HEALTH NURSING, ENVIRONMENTAL HEALTH PROGRAMS, AND HEALTH PROMOTION AND DISEASE PREVENTION. OUR PROGRAMS FOR IMMUNIZATIONS, ADOLESCENT SERVICES, AND WOMEN'S HEALTH HAVE RECEIVED NATIONAL RECOGNITION. IN SHIPROCK, 95% OF OUR CHILDREN ARE IMMUNIZED BECAUSE THE IHS AND TRIBAL PROGRAMS WORK TOGETHER WITH FAMILIES.

NO MATTER WHAT DECISIONS ARE MADE ON STAFFING AND FUNDING, IT IS CLEAR THAT THE HEALTH NEEDS OF OUR NAVAJO PEOPLE WILL NOT GO AWAY AND WILL NEED TO BE MET SOMEHOW.

FOR THE PAST TEN YEARS, THE SPECIALIZED MEDICAL SERVICES PROVIDED BY IHS WAS RECOGNIZED BY CONGRESS AND EXEMPTED IT FROM FEDERAL CEILINGS ON FULL TIME EQUIVALENT POSITIONS. IN FY '94, THE EXEMPTION WAS RESCINDED AND IHS WAS INCLUDED IN THE CEILINGS, AND IN FACT, INSTRUCTED TO REDUCE ITS OVERALL STAFFING. EFFORTS TO MEET CURRENT CEILINGS, AND FURTHER REDUCTIONS TO MEET THE PRESIDENT'S GOALS, WILL RESULT IN A LOSS OF ABOUT 85 POSITIONS FROM SHIPROCK SERVICE UNIT. THIS WILL ONLY WORSEN THE IMBALANCE OF NEEDS AND RESOURCES.

WE HEAR FROM " WASHINGDOON" THAT CUTS IN FUNDING AND STAFFING

ARE ONLY IN THE FUTURE. I AM HERE TO LET YOU KNOW THAT THEY ARE HAPPENING RIGHT NOW. WE ARE TOLD THAT CUTS "WILL NOT AFFECT THE HEALTH PROVIDERS" BUT, THE HIRING FREEZE FOR THE PAST FIVE MONTHS RESULTED IN LOSING DENTISTS, DOCTORS, AND NURSES WHO WANTED TO COME AND WORK IN SHIPROCK. JUST THIS MONTH, 13 EMPLOYEES RECEIVED TERMINATION NOTICES FOR "BUDGET REASONS". THESE PEOPLE PROVIDED DIRECT SERVICES INCLUDING AN OB NURSE, 2 MENTAL HEALTH COUNSELORS, 2 HEALTH EDUCATORS, 1 WOMEN'S HEALTH OUTREACH WORKER, AND OTHER SUPPORT PERSONNEL. THIS IS ONLY THE FIRST ROUND OF CUTS AND IT HAS ALREADY HAD A SIGNIFICANT NEGATIVE IMPACT ON PATIENT CARE AND FAMILY SERVICES.

OUR POPULATION AND OUR NEEDS ARE GROWING, SO WE NEED MORE STAFF, NOT LESS. THE IHS METHODOLOGY CALCULATES A NEED FOR 515 NEW POSITIONS. WE KNOW THIS NEED IS REAL.

THE RESOURCES TO PAY FOR THE NEW STAFF IS ABOUT $23 MILLION PER YEAR. EVEN WITH THIS INCREASE, SHIPROCK WILL SPEND $990 PER PERSON WHICH IS STILL BELOW THE OVERALL IHS AVERAGE OF $1,132, AND ONLY ONE FOURTH (1/4) OF THE NATIONAL HEALTH CARE SPENDING OF $3,760 PER PERSON.

WE NEED RELIEF FROM FEDERAL EMPLOYMENT CEILINGS, REDUCTION PLANS AND BUDGET CUTS. WE WANT TO FOLLOW THROUGH ON PLANS TO BRING A WIDER RANGE OF SERVICES CLOSER TO OUR PEOPLE, IN A MORE RESPECTFUL MANNER, WITH MORE REASONABLE WAITING TIMES.

WE WANT TO MAINTAIN THE PROGRESS WE ARE MAKING IN COMMUNITY AND PREVENTIVE HEALTH SERVICES. THESE PROGRAMS REALIZE SAVINGS IN THE LONG RUN.

LAST BUT NOT LEAST, WE REQUEST FOR LANGUAGE IN THE APPROPRIATION THAT THE 515 NEW POSITIONS AND FUNDS BE SPECIFICALLY EARMARKED FOR SHIPROCK. WE ARE AFRAID THAT IHS WILL USE THE NEW POSITIONS AND FUNDS TO REDUCE ITS FTE AND BUDGET REDUCTION AND EVEN ALLOCATE THE NEW POSITIONS TO OTHER IHS PROGRAMS. IF REDUCTIONS ARE TO OCCUR, IT SHOULD HAPPEN AT IHS HEADQUARTERS LEVEL. WE HAVE TOO MANY CHIEFS AND NOT ENOUGH INDIANS.

MR. CHAIRMAN, THIS CONCLUDES MY STATEMENT. WE WILL SUBMIT OUR MORE DETAILED BRIEFING BOOK FOR YOUR REVIEW AND RECORD. I WOULD BE HAPPY TO ANSWER ANY QUESTIONS YOU MAY HAVE FOR US.

WE ARE PLANNING OUR DEDICATION ON SEPTEMBER 2, 1994. GENTLEMEN, YOU ARE INVITED TO COME CELEBRATE WITH US.

BRIEFING BOOK

On

Impact of Proposed Reductions of Staffing and Funding for Shiprock Service Unit, Navajo Area Indian Health Service

SUMMARY

Planned cuts in staffing and funding for the new Shiprock Indian Health Service Hospital will have a devasting impact on the health of over 45,000 Navajo People. These cuts are being made from a "bare-bones" health care system that is already funded at only 1/8th of the national per capita level. These cuts will mean even longer waiting time to receive even less services from a brand new hospital that will stand half empty because of the lack of adequate staffing. They could also mean an end to successful community outreach and health promotion programs.

In the early 1980's, both the Navajo Nation and the Indian Health Service realized that IHS would not provide needed medical services in the current overcrowded Shiprock Hospital facility. The only way IHS could fulfill its obligation was to provide a larger space with additional staff. The planning documents, Program Justification Document and Program of Requirement, confirmed these shortages and IHS/PHS/DHHS approved the justification for a replacement hospital.

The U.S. Congress also recognized and agreed with IHS and therefore approved funds for a replacement hospital with additional staffing to provide the needed medical care that were lacking. By its approval, the U.S. Government obligated itself to fulfill these needs. Over $40 million was spent to construct a new hospital.

The new Northern Navajo Medical Center is 75% complete and is projected to open September 1994. The President's Executive Order to reduce federal employees adversely affects what Congress had intended for the Navajos. The impact of no new staffing would result in the new facility not being utilized to the maximum benefit. The level of services currently provided in the old existing hospital would remain the same despite the availability of a new and expanded hospital.

The IHS staffing methodology identified 515 additional positions to adequately staff the new facility. The cost to fund the 515 full-time positions is $23,610,175. There are also no funds identified for the activation costs. Activation costs include the move in expenses and the bare minimum requested by the Shiprock Service Unit is $700,000.

The Shiprock Service Unit is the largest service unit on the largest reservation in the United States. It provides comprehensive health services to 45,000 people, while being funded at only 1/8 of the national level. Despite lack of resources, there have been many accomplishments. The following briefing paper provides background information on the impact of the FTE cutbacks.

The DHHS, on behalf of the government, is reneging on its obligation by refusing to provide the necessary staffing to operate the new facility and provide comprehensive health care. We, therefore, strongly recommend that the government keep its promise and commitment to provide medical services and not use budgetary maneuvering to deny the Navajos the appropriate health care owed them.

The new Shiprock Hospital (Northern Navajo Medical Center) should be allowed to hire up to 515 additional staff, and $23,610,175 in additional funds added to the IHS budget to cover the cost of these new employees.

Planned cuts in staffing and funding for the new Shiprock Indian Health Service Hospital will have a devasting impact on the health of over 45,000 Navajo People. These cuts are being made from a"bare-bones" health care system that is already funded at only 1/8th of the national per capita level. These cuts will mean even longer waiting time to receive even less services from a brand new hospital that will stand half empty because of the lack of adequate staffing. They could also mean an end to successful community outreach and health promotion programs.

The Shiprock Service Unit of the Navajo Area Indian Health Service is the largest service unit on the largest reservation in the country, providing services to over 45,000 Native Americans living over a 5,000 square mile area in the Four Corners region of New Mexico, Arizona, Utah and Colorado.

During 1994, a new hospital will open in Shiprock, but recent funding cutbacks and cuts in staffing will prevent this new facility from being able to meet the growing health care needs of our expanding population. Caught between the dreams of increased services under health care reform, and the realities of reductions in the federal deficit and federal workforce, the new Shiprock hospital is in danger of becoming a cruel joke on the many patients and families who rely on the IHS as a partner in their health care.

Limitations on space, staffing and resources despite a growing population with increasing health needs have made the new facility a necessity. By working together with tribal health programs, traditional healers and community members, the Shiprock Service Unit has achieved impressive results in prevention and in clinical services. These accomplishments are threatened by new plans to open the new facility without any additional staffing. There are even plans to cut the current staff, even though the increasing needs have been well documented.

This briefing book is intended to provide decision makers with background information on the impact of these plans. Numbers, charts and statistics do not convey the most important information, however - that is contained in the stories told by our people. We urge those who are in a position to make decisions affecting our lives to take the time to listen to our real life stories and to our leaders.

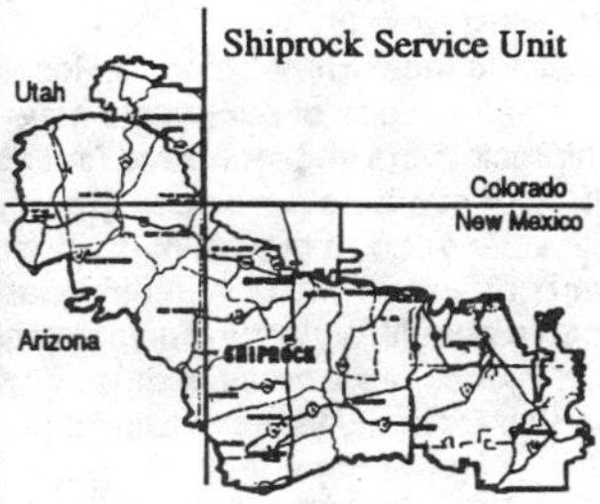

+

No new staffing

=

...will not be able to meet current needs

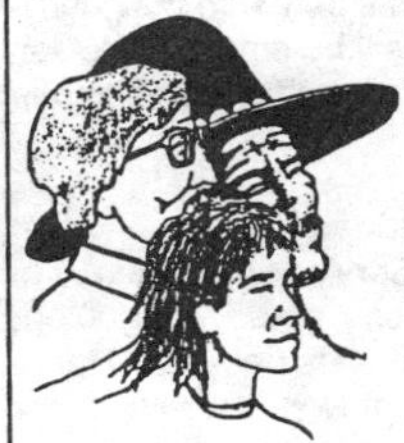

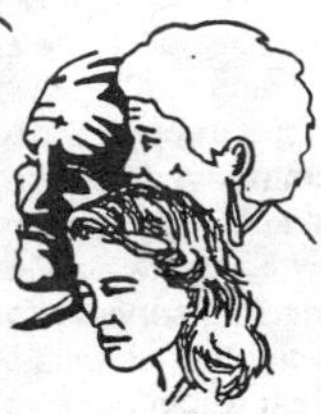

Key points: Shiprock Service Unit provides comprehensive health services, while needs continue to grow. Health services are underfunded (about 1/8 national level). Despite lack of resources, there have been many accomplishments. FTE reductions, and the lack of new staffing for the new Shiprock Hospital threaten the service unit's ability to meet population's health needs. Additional staffing and resources are sorely needed.

Growing Needs

Since the current Shiprock Hospital opened in 1959, the health needs of our people have continued to grow. Shiprock is the largest Native American community in the US. Our numbers have been growing at approximately 2.2% per year. About 1/2 of our population is under 20 years of age. We face increasing rates of diseases related to "Western lifestyles" including diabetes, heart disease and injuries. As a result of these growing needs, we have worked for many years to bring a new hospital to our area.

% of Population under 20

USA	Shiprock
28.6%	**47.3%**

In 1972 over $1 million dollars was spent to design a new Shiprock hospital. No money was ever set aside for construction. Community members, tribal leaders and the IHS staff did not give up, and after many years of hard work, our new Northern Navajo Medical Center is scheduled to open in Fall of 1994. Over $51 million was spent to construct a new 75 bed hospital, bringing us up to 1.6 beds per thousand people, as compared with a national rate of about 4.2 per thousand.

Hospital beds per 100 population

USA	**4.2**
Shiprock (current)	**1.1**
Shiprock (new)	**1.6**

BUT

Without additional staff, we will not be able to open all 75 beds. The IHS nursing staff feel they can only operate about 40 beds safely with their current level of staffing, so many rooms will be empty at the same time many of our people have to be shipped off to hospitals far away.

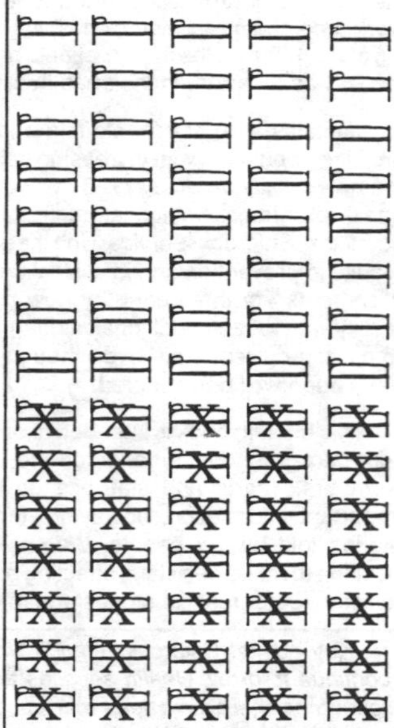

Without new staff, will only be able to safely operate 40 beds

Current Workload

Shiprock Service Unit is a very busy place, with over 3000 admissions, about 140,000 outpatient visits, and 900-1000 deliveries per year. Trends have been increasing in outpatient workload, while inpatient admissions have dropped because available beds have been limited due to nursing staffing issues. Over 50,000 of the outpatient visits come through the walk-in clinic or "treatment room" - a cramped, noisy room with two exam tables that can see over 300 patients on a busy winter day.

Shiprock Service Unit is the main source of health and medical services for most of our patients. When compared with other service units, more of our workload is people from within our own service unit, and a higher percentage of our service unit residences use our facilities for their care. 86% of the facility's inpatient workload is from Shiprock Service Unit residents. 92% of the facility's outpatient workload is from Shiprock Service Unit residents.

Funding

While national attention has been focussed on rapidly increasing health care expenditures, Shiprock Service Unit funding has not increased. Currently, the service unit is expected to provide comprehensive health care and public health services for less than $500 per person per year, compared with 1993 national expenditures of $3760 per year and 1992 expenditures of over $3200 per Medicare patient.

US Health Expenditures have been going up while Shiprock stays the same

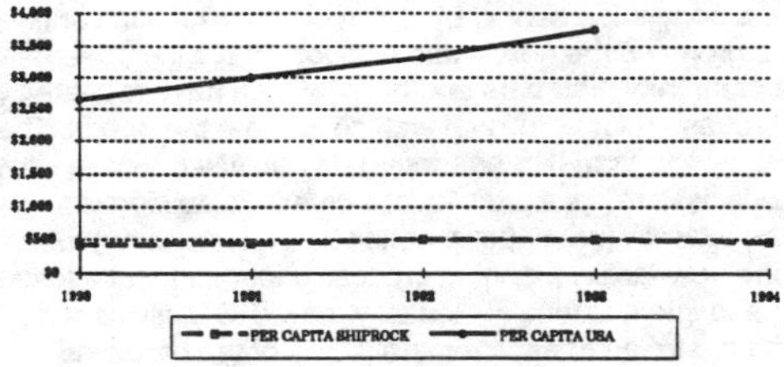

When compared with other federal direct care programs, the differences are even more glaring. While there are over 26 million veterans in America, only 2.8 million are eligible for VA medical care. This compares with 1.9 million American Indians noted in the 1990 census. With a medical care budget of over $16 billion in the President's FY 95 budget, the VA has over $5750 per eligible veteran to spend on health care. By contrast, the Indian Health Service has just over $1000 per person per year. In fact the 1.3 billion dollar increase in the VA budget [with about 500 million for increased health services] is just about the same size as the *entire* IHS clinical services budget. A 1992 GAO report showed Navajo Area to be below average at $775 per capita per year.

	<u>VA</u>	<u>IHS</u>
# eligible for health care	2.8 million	1.9 million
Health Budget	$16 billion	$2 billion
Per Capita	$5,750	$1,132
Navajo Area IHS Per capita		*$775*
Shiprock Service Unit Per Capita		***$489***

With the largest population of any Navajo Area Service Unit, Shiprock is funded at an even lower level. **The 1994 recurring allowance of $10.3 million amounts to only $226 per capita.** After figuring in Contract Health costs as well as Medicare / Medicaid and Private Insurance Collections, Shiprock Service Unit has about $489 per person to spend during FY 94 for comprehensive health care.

Within Navajo Area, Shiprock ranks #1 in population, #2 in clinical workload, but only #4 in funding, and #6 in per capita funding [1993 data. In 1994, allowance for Shiprock is even less]

Shiprock's Ranking Within Navajo Area IHS

Population	**#1**
Workload	**#2**
Funding	**#4**
Per Capita $	**#6**

Shiprock is #1 in Population

US Census Indian Population	
Shiprock #1	***43,311***
Gallup	28,808
Ft. Defiance	27,529
Chinle	27,515
Tuba City	25,539
Kayenta	16,447
Crownpoint	16,301
Winslow	14,386

Shiprock is #2 in Outpatient Visits

Outpatient Visits	
Gallup	198,975
Shiprock #2	***139,064***
Chinle	128,501
Tuba City	106,335
Ft. Defiance	81,358
Kayenta	69,271
Crownpoint	50,678
Winslow	47,414

Shiprock is #4 in In Clinical Funding

Clinical Funding	
Gallup	$30,929,587
Chinle	$23,730,656
Tuba City	$19,792,600
Shiprock #4	***$19,350,064***
Ft. Defiance	$11,200,436
Crownpoint	$ 8,502,479
Kayenta	$ 5,934,275
Winslow	$ 4,440,574

Shiprock is #6 in Funding Per Capita

Per Capita [1993]	
Gallup	$1,342
Chinle	$ 990
Tuba City	$ 988
Ft. Defiance	$ 690
Crownpoint	$ 679
Shiprock #6	***$ 590***
Kayenta	$ 483
Winslow	$ 479

Shiprock Steering Committee Briefing Book 3/3/94

Staffing

Since plans for a new hospital were cancelled in 1972, the population served by Shiprock Hospital has continued to grow. As the needs and workload have increased, community members and hospital staff have repeatedly requested for additional staffing to meet the needs. The response from IHS headquarters has always been - *the only way to get a significant increase in staffing is to get a new facility* [no matter that needs are increasing] In fact, the new facility planning process attempts to take levels of need into account. Historically, new IHS facilities have been staffed at approximately 85% of the projected need - with the increases sometimes spaced out over two years - called "annualization".

Several estimates of the need for increased staffing have been calculated based on IHS planning formulae (RRMNA) which are undergoing revision. Initial calculations showed a need for 264 additional staff positions. Some of the early budget plans for the IHS took this into account, with calls for 170 additional positions for Shiprock in the FY 95 budget. This number was reduced 10/12 to 142 because headquarters felt staff would not be hired until one or two months in to FY 95. Recalculations of need, based on "new RRMNA nursing modules" which more accurately reflect nursing needs for safe care, have led to estimates of need as high as 515 positions to safely operate the new facility. The Administration's budget for FY 95 calls for NO NEW POSITIONS for Shiprock.

Shiprock Hospital will be the first new IHS facility *ever* to open without any increase in staffing.

In fact Government -wide plans for reduction in the size of the federal workforce (called FTE reduction) call for reductions in staffing of as many as 105 positions from the current staffing at Shiprock Service Unit.

FTE reduction is being unfairly applied to Indian Health Service - they are being asked to take more than twice their fair share of cuts. Perhaps this is because decision-makers feel there will be little political cost in cutting such a program unfairly. In fact several "vital" programs within DHHS appear to be increasing in staff size during the FTE reduction. With 11.9% of the DHHS staff working within IHS, they are being asked to take on more than 25% of the department-wide reduction.

National Comparisons:

Number of People Served per Physician

USA	**416**
Shiprock	**1,500**

Number of People Served per Psychiatrist

USA	**5,555**
State of NM	**5,700**
Shiprock	**22,905**

Estimates of the new staff needed:

RRMNA initial value -	**264**
IHS HQ annualized need -	**170**
IHS HQ 10/12 cut -	**142**
New RRMNA modules-	**515**
President's Budget -	**0**

Total Funds needed for 515 additional positions = **$23,610,175**

FTE reduction - **cut by 105**

Total IHS FTE's FY 1993 : **15,418**

This is **11.9%** of DHHS total FTE's

Total FTE reduction for IHS - **1,289**
Total FTE reduction for DHHS **-5,200**

IHS is absorbing more than 25% of the total departmental reduction - more than twice it's "fair share":

Impact of "no new positions" or staff cuts with the new hospital

Outpatient Care Improvements will be impossible. Neither the staff nor the patients feel good about the rushed, crowded "doc-in-the-box" approach used in the treatment room. Responding to concerns from the community health board, staff have developed a plan for improved outpatient care that would - increase chances of seeing "your own doctor" [not just whoever is on call], provide much more scheduled appointment time for family medicine services, shorten waiting times considerably, change the focus from the immediate problem to more comprehensive care, and allow patients to be seen in their own doctor's office, rather than the walk-in area. Without new nursing staff, these plans will be impossible to achieve and the new hospital will become just a bigger waiting area - with longer waits for the same rushed, impersonal care from a different doctor every time, without much attention to the ongoing chronic medical problems of the patient.

Plans to address Common Problems:

- **Long Waits**
- **Lack of Continuity**
- **Impersonal Care**

......will be impossible to implement

Specific New Services that will be impacted:

We are very glad to have a **CT scanner** in our new facility, which will benefit patients from all over the reservation. However, without new X-ray staffing, either no one will be able to operate it, or we will have to cut down on our "regular" x-ray procedures like ultrasounds and routine x-rays (which are already so overbooked we often have to wait several weeks to schedule and ultrasound or special x-ray test).

- **Forced to choose - leave CT scanner turned off, or cut back on other x-ray services**

Our people need access to the new specialized surgery services with an **orthopedist, ENT surgeon, and urologist** on staff. However without additional nursing staff, their services will be very limited. We will only be able to operate 2 of the 4 operating rooms.

- **May only open two of four operating rooms**

More space to clean with **no additional housekeeping staff.** Already they are so busy they can only clean some areas once a week.

- **Who will keep the new hospital clean - will sick patients have to clean their own rooms?**

More square footage to maintain, and complicated new computer controlled utility systems in the new hospital - **without any additional maintenance staff** means our patients won't benefit from the improvements as the limited staff have to deal with crisis problems.

- **Room by room climate control is nice but need maintenance staff to operate it. Many new systems in new hospital - may fail without additional staff**

Shiprock Steering Committee Briefing Book 3/3/94

Existing Programs That will be Impacted

Rural Health Stations and Health Centers in Sanostee, Toadlena and Teec Nos Pos may be among the first to go, making health care less accessible for some of those most in need.

• Cuts in services available to remote areas

Contracting for dietary or housekeeping services would result in many jobs lost for local, skilled Navajo workers.

• Loss of local jobs

Current weaknesses, especially waiting times, will be worsened.

• Old problems just get worse

We may lose specific services like diabetes care, eye care or special care unit.

• Specific services may be lost

Our service unit commitment to prevention may be questioned, as "life threatening" emergencies and crises take up most of our funding and staff. With reduced resources, it would make sense to increase our commitment to prevention, but the clinical pressures to cut prevention in order to maintain medical services will be intense.

• Threatens our commitment to prevention - may lose progress on immunizations, adolescent care

Staffing cutbacks threaten our comprehensive system of care. The automatic referral of all newborns for a public health nurse home visit; the commitment of resources to immunization efforts; the linkage between primary care and counseling services for adolescents; easy access to high quality social services - all will be jeopardized but the planned staffing cutbacks in the face of growing population and growing need.

• Loss of comprehensive care

Contracting for Services is generally not a viable option in Shiprock. For many services -such as dental care -there is no available "pool" of contractors. Our experience with contracting for clinical services is that nursing or medical contractors cost 2 to 3 times as much as our own staff. Using contractors to meet FTE reduction requirements will result in increased costs - without any increase in our budget, this will force us to cut services even further.

Average incomes

MD at Shiprock	$ 80,000
MD in US	$165,000
Contract MD cost	$200,000

The Navajo Tribal Government is well aware of its right to request to operate the entire program under "638" legislation. They are also aware however, that to undertake such a project without significantly increased resources is a course that is destined to fail. The problem of inadequate resources to meet growing needs will not be solved by transferring the operating responsibility while continuing to fund the program at 1/8 the national rate of expenditures.

• Problem is lack of adequate resources to meet the needs. If Navajo Tribe chooses to operate hospital, or if IHS continues to operate - either way additional resources are the key

Activation Costs

The costs of moving patients, beds, equipment, supplies and over 400 staff members to the new facility are significant. It has been the usual practice of the IHS to budget "activation costs" for new facilities. Shiprock PHS administrative staff have developed plans for activation activities and related costs several times over the past two years. With each new set of instructions from headquarters, the amount planned for is reduced. At the current time NO MONEY FOR ACTIVATION OR MOVING COSTS IS INCLUDED in either the FY 94 or 95 budgets. They are even exploring the possibility of using the National Guard to help move to the new facility. Without activation funding, any move to the new facility will have to be funded out of the hospital's already limited operating budget, and will result in further decreases in services for our people

IHS has historically provided "start-up" and moving costs with new facilities to keep these costs from cutting into operating budgets.

The initial estimate from 2/93 included:

- temporary staff,
- overtime for current staff involved in moving
- 6 permanent staff [to hire "early" to facilitate ordering equipment, hiring staff, overseeing move process]
- Rentals and storage space
- Commercial moving company
- New linens
- Maintenance supplies needed for new facility
- Utility costs for one month overlap of two facilities
- Transportation costs

Estimated Activation Costs calculated 2/4/93: **$2,964,750**

The staff were told to revise their estimate downward and on 2/11/94 submitted a "bare bones plan", eliminating any additional staffing, cutting back on overtime, no new linens, a 90% reduction in maintenance supplies, no contracts for activation, and the elimination of most transportation and storage expenses.

Revised "Bare Bones" Activation Costs Request: **$700,039**

The ideas that we would open a new hospital, but can't afford new linens for the beds, or that we could spend over $51 million for a new hospital but can't use it because we can't afford to move across the street have led to intense community concern.

AMOUNT BUDGETED IN FY 94

$0

AMOUNT BUDGETED IN FY 95

$0

IMPACT - FURTHER CUTS IN SERVICES OR NO MOVE

Shiprock Steering Committee Briefing Book 3/3/94

Needs are increasing

Shiprock Service Unit's population is growing at over 2% per year. Median age is 22. Birth rate is twice the national average.

About 20% of children are born to teenage mothers, leading to increased demands on the social service and school systems. Functioning extended family networks, in many cases, result in better outcomes for teen pregnancy in our area, when compared with national levels

In the 1960's researchers studied why Navajo people did not get heart disease, searching for a "protective factor". By the 1990's rates of heart disease among our men have caught up to the national levels, and are continuing to increase while national rates are falling.

The impact of diabetes is growing with more and more of our people on dialysis machines and losing their legs or their eyesight. It has only been in the past two or three years that we have begun to see children with diabetes among our people.

We are seeing increasing numbers of injuries due to interpersonal violence including child abuse, child sexual abuse, partner abuse and elder abuse. Our homicide and suicide rates are high. Surveys of public school students in grades 4-12 show that 22% report having been injured with a weapon in the past 12 months.

Injuries, illness and family problems related to alcohol and drugs continue to affect our communities, just as they do the rest of the country.

Trauma is the number one cause of mortality. This drives a need for trauma care (ER, Surgical, ICU, orthopedic care), as well as injury prevention and alcohol treatment programs

Rodent population related disease are rare but result in high case fatality rate

These needs are not going to go away. Whatever the level of cutbacks, the staff of Shiprock Service Unit will have to try and meet these needs, in cooperation with tribal programs, community members and traditional healers.

- Birth rate US -16, Navajo - 29
- Population grew 24% between 1980 and 1990 census
- Special needs of children and teen populations
- High volume of prenatal care, family planning, immunizations, well child care
- Teen Pregenancy accounts for 20% of deliveries

- Rates of heart disease among Navajo people have "caught up" to national rates.

Shiprock Service Unit
- 10/8 -9/90 **31 amputations in 4 yrs**
- 1/93-12/93 **40 amputations in 1 yr**

On Dialysis
CY '90 - **61** patients
CY '93 - **76** patients
(61% due to diabetes)

% reporting having been injured with a weapon in previous 12 months - Grades 4-12, Shiprock Area Public Schools
1990 - **24%**
1992 - **22%**

- Alcohol - related problems

- Trauma is leading cause of death

- Hantavirus, plague are important

Partners in healing

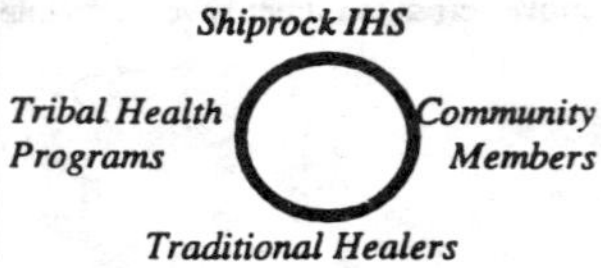

Shiprock Steering Committee Briefing Book 3/3/94

Other Local resources are limited

Percent Unemployed (1990)		Median Household Income		Percent Below Poverty Level	
US	6.3 %	US	$30,056	US	13.1 %
American Indian/ Alaska Native (all US)	15.4 %	American Indian/ Alaska Native (all US)	$19,865	American Indian/ Alaska Native (all US)	31.7 %
Navajo Nation	27.9 %	Navajo Nation	$10,433	Navajo Nation	56.1 %

• Lack of communication and transportation complicates health care delivery and follow up - this impacts clinic visits, surgery and patient teaching efforts.
• Lack of indoor plumbing causes a large urgent care volume of gastrointestinal and respiratory illness, and makes it difficult to car for illness at home [after hauling water for 40 miles, our diabetic patients are unlikely to" waste" it on soaking their feet daily]
• Relation between poverty and health status is well established.

Household Information

• 78% of homes have no telephones
• 54% of homes have no electricity
• 52% of homes have no indoor plumbing
•26% of occupied housing units have no vehicle, and public transportation is very limited

• Tribal health programs work well together with IHS, community groups at the local level. This is evident in the close relationships between CHR's and Public Health Nurses, TB workers and Chest Clinic doctors, Health Education staff and IHS Community Health Service staff, and WIC and MCH clinic staff.

• WIC has limited funding - much less than the need
•IHS Needs Assessment methodology shows need for 44 CHR's within Shiprock Service Unit - there are only 14 due to lack of funding
•Tribal alcohol program not able to pay for inpatient rehab except in rare cases

Community Resources are a vital part of the health service "team",
Just a few examples at right...

• Schools - Public and BIA
• Law Enforcement and Judicial
• Women's Shelter
• Local board operates adolescent treatment center in Shiprock

Traditional teachings have great power in prevention efforts. Likewise, traditional healers work together with IHS and tribal health workers to bring our patients back into balance. Many patients seek spiritual wellness or healing through traditional Navajo medicine, the Native American Church, and through Christian churches.

• Spiritual healing and wellness are parts of community spectrum of services.

78-786 - 94 - 3

Shiprock Steering Committee Briefing Book 3/3/94

Program accomplishments

Immunization rates consistently > 90%

Despite challenges proposed by a remote rural area with poor access to transportation, dirt roads, and a very few telephones for follow-up, Shiprock Service Unit has made childhood immunization a priority. As a result of hard work by the Public Health Nurses, Maternal and Child Health Clinic, and concern parents and grandparents, we have consistently achieved immunization rates over 90% for the past 10 years. The capacity of the system was tested by a measles outbreak in 1991 on the other side of the reservation. Within two weeks, Shiprock staff have immunized over 10,000 people with their second dose of MMR vaccine. As a result there were no confirmed cases in the Shiprock area of the reservation.

Strategic planning, involves community members

Since 1990, Shiprock Service Unit has been involved in a community based strategic planning initiative which focuses on concerns of local staff and local community members. Goals are set in four areas of excellence and planning efforts include full participation by the 20 members of the Shiprock area community health board.

Adolescent Health Services

There are over 10,000 adolescents between the ages of 10 - 19 in Shiprock Service Unit. Targeted services have been developed since 1987 including establishment of an adolescent health center at Teen Life Center and 7 area high schools and middle schools. The center provides primary health care, prenatal care, and group, individual and family counseling services. The center has already had a significant impact on utilization of prenatal care services and rates of school completion among pregnant teens. Over the past several years counseling services have focused on school support groups, peer based mediation, development of a young people's AA group and operation of an experiential therapy ropes course.

Women's Health Project

A cooperative effort with the State of New Mexico and Centers for Disease Control and Prevention has resulted in increased availability of preventive health services for women. Prior to the initiations of the project there was no screening mammography available through the IHS system. There has been a high level of acceptance of preventive services including mammography since they have been made available and more accessible to people at the local level by bringing these services to the rural health stations and health centers. Significant improvements have been shown in rate of mammography, rate of BSE teaching and rate of pap smears. During the first year of the Women's Health Project 12 early breast cancers were found. The Women's Health Project also includes a significant outreach portion with community based focus groups and preventive health education. During the first two years of the statewide project, Shiprock did over 23% of the work done in the entire state even though they were only one of 65 project sites!

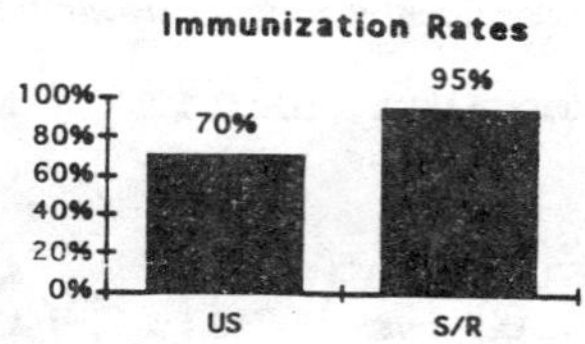

Financial coverage for immunizations

•Employer based insurance	45
•Preferred provider organization	62
•Health maintenance organizations	98
•Shiprock PHS	100

CUSTOMER SERVICE

CLINICAL SERVICES — *EXCELLENCE* — *MANAGEMENT*

HEALTH PROMOTION

Prenatal Care for Pregnant Teens

	% with late (3rd trimester) or no care	% with 1st trimester care
1987	55%	15%
1990	25%	35%
1993		45%

began in-school service in '87-'88 school year

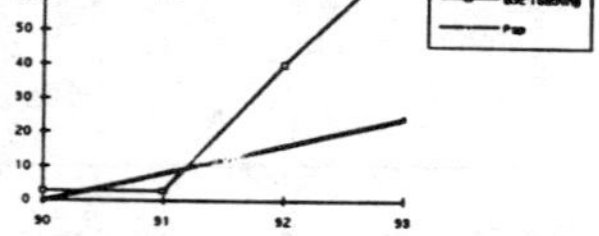

•Increased services by additional staff, evening clinics, using outlying clinics, outreach education program.

Diabetes Program

Just now starting to see children with Diabetes
Amputation, dialysis rates increasing markedly

Shiprock Service Unit Diabetes Program provides clinical and educational services to 2,600 diabetic patients and their families.

- 150 to 180 Diabetic Pts a year • new pts visit DM Clinic monthly
  - education - Community exercise program
  - support group - evening DM Clinic for working pts
  - clinical care - summer camp for children of DM pts
  - In its 7th year, exercise program has > 60 instructors trained

Audiovisual education materials

The Health Promotion Department together with the clinical and nurse departments have produced many culturally specific Navajo language materials for patient education. In addition weekly Navajo language radio spots on health issues are aired over local radio stations. Materials are also developed by working together with community groups addressing health issues of local concern.

Seasonal messages

A coordinated community and clinic based approach to nutrition and exercise teaching has begun in fiscal year 1994. This approach includes community education with radio PSA's, billboards and grocery store based education together with reinforced messages from the clinic. A different set of messages is organized for each season. These messages are organized among the four directions of Navajo tradition philosophy. During the spring '94 message, patients with chronic disease such as diabetes and hypertension will not only be urged to eat more fruits and vegetables, but will be provided with seeds and information about water resources and gardening through a cooperative agreement with Navajo Department of Agriculture.

Focus on injury prevention

Injuries are the leading cause of mortality among Navajos aged 0 to 44. Motor vehicle crashes are the leading cause of injury fatalities. Other injury fatalities have resulted from homicide, suicide and drowning. With injuries as a leading cause of death among young adults both on the reservation and the US, specific efforts at injury prevention have been underway for several years in Shiprock Service Unit. Safety education and injury prevention campaigns have resulted in a decrease in the rate of morbidity and mortality due to injuries in the Shiprock Service Unit and we have also seen significant increases in the rate of seat belt use, decreases in the rate of fatal motor vehicle crashes and serious MVA requiring ER visits. Current injury prevention efforts focus on prevention of pedestrian injuries related to alcohol and prevention of interpersonal intentional injuries including domestic violence. These efforts involve cooperative arrangements with State, Tribal and local community resources. The IHS is the major and a very important artner in these efforts.

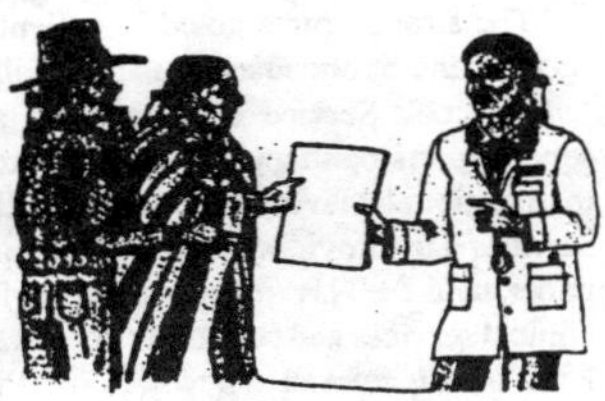

24 Videos Completed by Health Promotion in FY'93
Examples:

- **Singing Eyes**
  Laser Treatment for Patients with Diabetes
- **Beat Diabetes '93**
  Patient Panel from Diabetes Conference in Farmington, NM
- **Medical Records**
  It's not just the doctors who care for you
- **Construction Blues**
  New hospital construction music video
- **Back to School**
  Crosswalk awareness - traffic safety
- **Summertime Blues**
  Summer activities - Shiprock Youth Center summer schedule

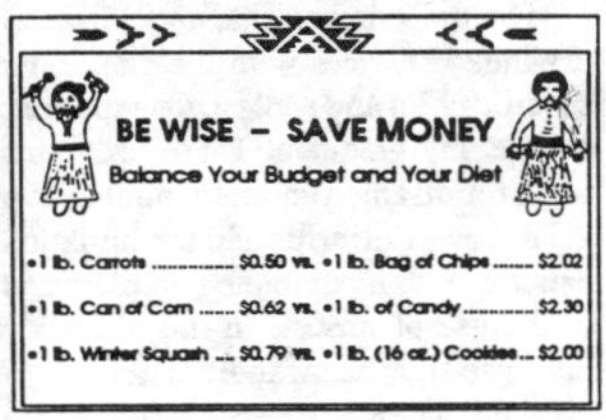
BE WISE – SAVE MONEY
Balance Your Budget and Your Diet
•1 lb. Carrots .... $0.50 vs. •1 lb. Bag of Chips $2.02
•1 lb. Can of Corn .... $0.62 vs. •1 lb. of Candy $2.30
•1 lb. Winter Squash ... $0.79 vs. •1 lb. (16 oz.) Cookies ... $2.00

Shiprock Service Unit Rates per 100,000 of Motor Vehicle Crashes leading to fatalities

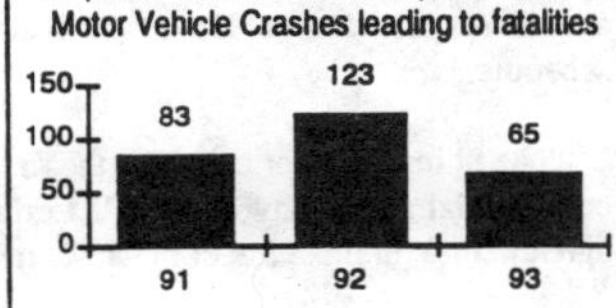

Shiprock Service Unit Rates per 100,000 of All Fatalities due to Injuries

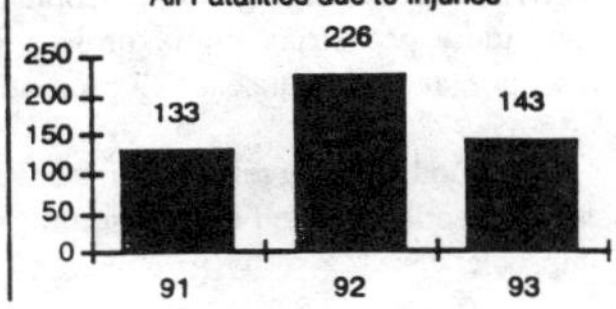

Strengths of our system, as perceived by Patients

The strong points noted in patient satisfaction surveys, staff surveys and public meetings are as follows:

Shiprock Service Unit provides a comprehensive range of service (one stop shopping), services are provided with a sensitivity to traditional Navajo culture as well as other cultural issues, services are provided with access to health professionals who understand the Navajo language, services include a link between clinical services and community based services (an example would be automatic referral of newborns for Public Health Nursing visits) , services focus on preventive as well as clinical services, and staff are seen as hard working, dedicated.

- **Comprehensive Services Package at one site**
- **Cultural Sensitivity**
- **Navajo language**
- **Integrate preventive services**
- **Committed staff**

Nursing /Clinical accomplishments

In the past several years nursing and clinical departments have developed special services in responses to community needs and program limitations. One specific example is a development of a day surgery program. This enables patients to get home sooner, relieving burdens on their families. This is coupled with an initiation of laparoscopic gallbladder surgery services in the past three years, has reduced inpatient stays for surgery significantly.

On the clinical side the Physical Therapy Department has expanded services with the addition of a physical therapist with specific child and adolescent experience, and a new Navajo physical therapy graduate. These programs include expansion of services for disabled children, pool therapy for patients with paraplegia or severe arthritis and the initiation of a "gaiting program" for patients with incomplete paraplegia, allowing them to walk again to the use of braces. In this specific case this specific program involved significant additional work for a physical therapy department but was required because IHS health contract services would not pay for outside gaiting programs. In order to provide the service to our patients physical therapists needed to locate outside resources to pay for the braces, and provide direct service for this additional program on top of their already overloaded clinical schedule.

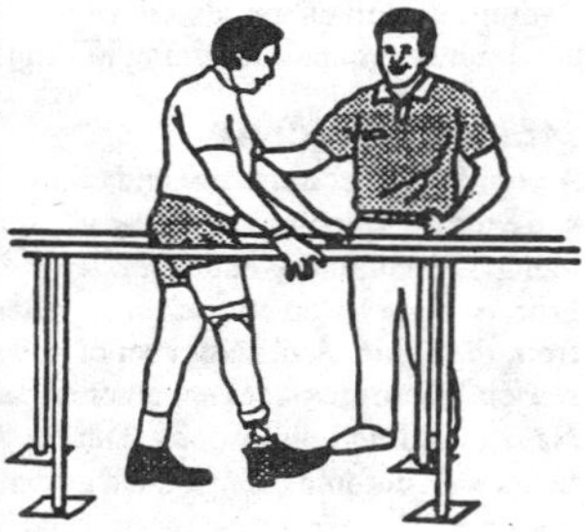

The Shiprock laboratory was the first NAIHS site to offer both confidential and anonymous HIV testing, through a cooperative agreement with the State of New Mexico, beginning in 1992.

- **First Anonymous HIV testing program in NAIHS**

The Nursing units have shown a strong commitment to community involvement and health promotion. Their staff have been involved in encouraging young people to choose health careers, a community pedestrian injury project, poison prevention, AIDS education and car seat/seat belt promotion, among other issues.

The good working relationship between physicians and nursing staff is frequently cited as a reason for nurses choosing to stay at Shiprock.

Recent Nursing Accomplishments

- **Markedly improved retention**
- **decrease in bedsores to zero**
- **Involvement in community**
- **Discharge Planning begun 1991**
- **Case Management model 1993**
- **Self governance of nursing units**
- **Nurse-managed diabetes clinic**
- **JCAHO accreditation**
- **Day Surgery Program**

Response to hantavirus outbreak showed strengths of comprehensive system, commitment of staff.

At the end of May 1993 a mysterious and deadly new disease appeared on the reservation. While the assistance of national resources such as the CDC were very important, the majority of public education, investigation and patient care services were provided through local, IHS and Tribal Health Program staff. Information updates were provided through radio and at community central points almost daily through the months of June and July 1993. A short video project addressing local fears and concerns as well as describing the clinical syndrome, was completed in 24 hours and distributed to all 20 local chapters within 2 days. The outbreak resulted in a doubling or tripling of outpatient workload, intensive care for extremely ill patients and dealing with communities that were frighten as well as somewhat angry with the national media attention and labeling of this as a "Navajo Illness". The local response of the IHS, Tribal Health staff and community leaders demonstrated the strengths of a comprehensive, community based system with the very committed staff. It is unlikely that this syndrome would have been identified as early, and that a coordinated local response could have been so quickly developed in a "fee for service" system.

Hantavirus Impact and Response
- Marked increase in clinical workload
- Community Fears
- Community education began immediately - constant updates
- Video project completed within a day and sent out to 20 communities.
- Close cooperation between local IHS & tribal health workers
- Media Impact negative

Other Communicable disease with Team Responses
- Measles outbreak - 10,000 immunizations given in one month
- Hepatitis A - school outbreaks
- Plague Team
- HIV prevention education, testing

Program weaknesses identified by patients

While most patients are satisfied with the care they receive, the number one concern is the long waiting time to receive care. Multiple "time studies have been done to identify bottlenecks in the system and many changes have been made to decrease waits, but the key problem remains lack of adequate staff and space to meet patient needs.

- **Waiting time is too long**

Very limited clinic space has led to a system where providers have very few "continuity clinics", and spend most of their time in walk-in and emergency care. Patients in these settings often see a different provider every visit. These visits often focus only on the immediate problem and the rushed format does not allow time for discussion of chronic problems, or more personal issues. These leads some patients to complain that care is "impersonal".

- **See a different provider every time - Why can't I see "my own doctor"?**
- **Care is too rushed**

When patients require services not available at Shiprock PHS, they use the "contract health" system - which is like a limited IHS insurance company. There are many restrictions on what types of services can be covered through contract care, and services are clearly rationed based on resources available and the urgency of need. Because resources are always very limited, contract care often only pays for emergency or life threatening conditions. Many other services, such as alcohol treatment, physical rehabilitation (except immediately after an injury), prosthetic dental work, non-emergent specialist consultation or referral - are not covered. Patients often complain about the confusing rules regarding contract coverage and when they are left with all or part of a bill from another provider.

- **Contract Care system is complicated.**
- **Many services are not covered by contract health - especially if they aren't life threatening.**

Shiprock Steering Committee Briefing Book 3/3/94

Comparison of our System with Washington, D.C.

Washington, DC is home to over 600,000 people, who spent over $2 billion on health care in 1992. For this money, what they got was over 150,000 people without health coverage, infant mortality rates of three or four times the national rate, and only about 1/2 of their children adequately immunized. All of this for a mere $3,300 per person.

In contrast, for under $500 per person, Shiprock Service Unit provides coverage for everyone, has reduced infant mortality to match national levels, and has demonstrated its commitment to children by making sure that more than 95% are fully immunized.

As government policy makers make decisions from far away that threaten our accomplishments and our access to care, our people have to wonder if the goal is to make us more like Washington, DC?

- **%of people with health coverage**

Washington DC	75%
Shiprock	100%

- **Infant mortality rate**

Washington DC	30-40
Shiprock	10.5

- **% Children fully immunized**

Washington DC	50%
Shiprock	95%

- **Per Capita Health Expenditures**

Washington DC	$3,300
Shiprock	$ 489

Basis of IHS services

While we have established that the needs are great and the resources limited, the basis for Indian Health Service's obligation to provide services is not that need, but rather solemn agreements between sovereign nations. Ours is a "prepaid" health care system, in which the payment was made many years ago in terms of land and the many sacrifices of our great grandparents.

- Not based on poverty or need, [though both are real] - but on treaty and trust obligations

The federal trust responsibility of the US government means that health services must be provided fairly and reasonably. To cut staff disproportionately from the IHS [while needs are growing], while at the same time expanding other programs - is not a fair or reasonable practice.

- Inequities in funding between IHS areas, and between IHS and other federal programs within DHHS do not appear to be fair or reasonable

Each of us is responsible for his or her own health choices, but the Indian Health Service is a vital part of our local resources.

- Patients and families rely on IHS to be there as a partner in their journeys toward wellness

Our system is far from perfect, but the rest of the country could learn something from our efforts:

- How to provide universal coverage at reasonable cost
- How to meet national immunization targets
- How to integrate prevention and health promotion into health services
- How to reduce infant mortality in "high risk" areas
- How to work together with communities, use lay health workers, and rely on family and community strengths.

- ***The rewards for these achievements seem to include staffing and funding cuts, while the rest of the country debates details about health insurance.***

The Problem

Planned cuts in staffing and funding for the new Shiprock Indian Health Service Hospital will have a devasting impact on the health of over 45,000 Navajo People. These cuts are being made from a "bare-bones" health care system that is already funded at only 1/8th of the national per capita level. These cuts will mean even longer waiting time to receive even less services from a brand new hospital that will stand half empty because of the lack of adequate staffing. They could also mean an end to successful community outreach and health promotion programs.

What is Needed

In order to address the growing needs of the largest service unit on the largest Indian Reservation in the United States, several things are needed:

•The new hospital must come with additional staffing in order to fully utilize the new facility, and even to be able to continue to provide the current limited services to our growing population.

•The cost of these new positions would be approximately $23 million. When added to current allowances, this would result in funding at a per capita level of only $990 - still below the IHS average of $1,132 per capita and well below the national health care spending level of $3,760 per person.

•Continued commitment to excellence in clinical services, management, health promotion and customer service. Cuts in staffing or funding should not be at the expense of patient care or community prevention efforts.

•Proposals to cut significantly from funding and staffing at the service unit levels at all IHS facilities should be re-examined. These cuts will have a devastating impact on the health status of the first Americans.

• 515 additional positions

• Additional funding of $23,610,175 to cover new positions

Per capita health funding

Current Shiprock $ 489

Shiprock with addtional positions $ 990

IHS average $1,132

USA Average $3,760

Muttonman by Vincent Craig

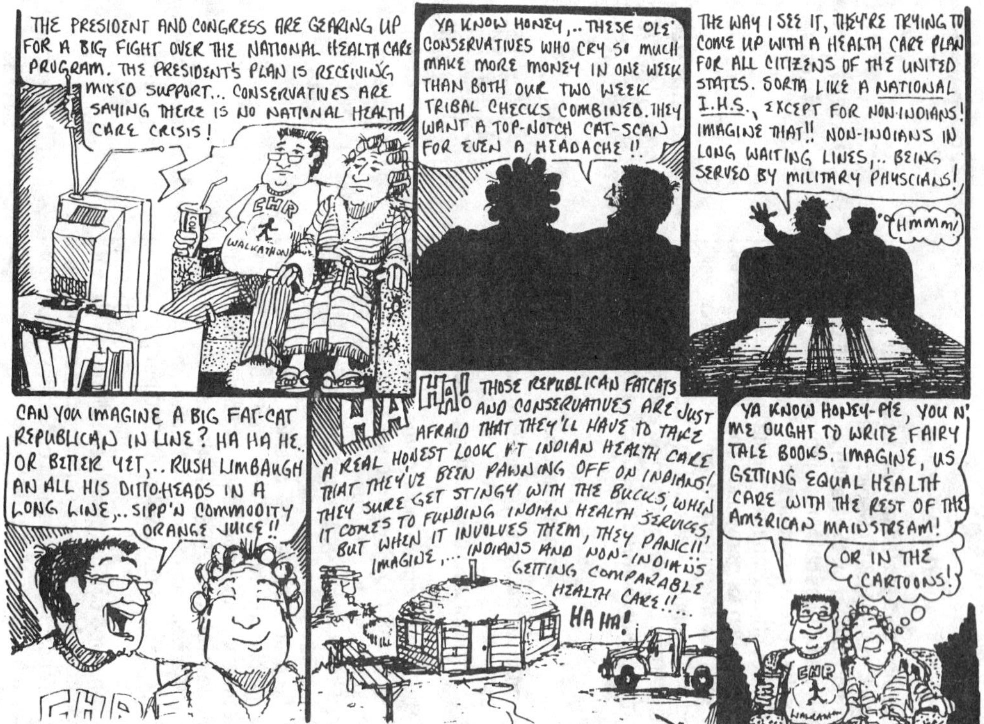

January 3, 1994

FROM: **Dee Hutchison, CEO-SRSU**

SUBJECT: **IMPACT OF FTE REDUCTION - SHIPROCK SERVICE UNIT**

TO: **Ron Wood , EO**

The following are prioritized options for FTE reductions, and their considerations and impacts.

Options:

1 - FURLOUGH

2 - TERMINATION OF TEMPORARY POSITIONS

3 - PERMANENT VACANT POSITIONS FREEZE AND/OR TERMINATION

4 - RESTRUCTURING OF DEPARTMENTS/PROGRAMS/SERVICES:

- **(a) Elimination of entire departments/programs/services.**
- **(b) Consolidation of departments/programs/services**
- **(c) Contracting services out to the private sector**

5 - 638 SELF DETERMINATION CONTRACTS

Considerations:

1. **Will furlough affect direct patient care positions or essential positions be exempted? Need to define essential positions.**

2. **No Commissioned Officers can be furlough.**

3. **Elapse time to implement furlough.**

4. **Union negotiations: employee rights, notification, and implementation of furlough.**

5. **Length of furlough (1 year, 2 years, etc.), and number of hours per employee per annum.**

6. **Length of temporary (filled) positions that are identified for termination need to be determined.**

7. Whether to terminate all temporary positions or retain essential temporary positions need to be determined.

8. Determining the type of permanent positions to freeze or eliminate without impeding patient care service will be a difficult task, because clinical services and support services are interdependent in operating a health care facility effectively and efficiently.

Impact:

1. Increased overtime and compensatory time to meet the workload when staff are on furlough status, termination and freezing of positions; hence, impacting the Service Unit Operating budgets.

2. Shifting of workload to staff who continue to work or delay in getting the job done due to shortage of personnel. Maybe some work just won't get accomplished. Most staff do more than their job descriptions. This action means added duties to already overworked staff, i.e., physicians are responsible for clinical and administrative duties, most support services are already understaffed, and clinical staff require support services.

3. Single employee offices will be closed during furlough.

4. When furloughing supervisors, lack of appropriate supervision of departments or programs.

5. Manpower and time are required to establish, implement, and supervise a well defined furlough schedule.

6. Economic impact on employees. Some employees live from paycheck to paycheck. Furlough and termination may cause financial burdens on such employees.

7. Employees' morale and quality of work may be greatly diminished because of furlough and termination of positions and employees. Is my job safe? Will I be terminated? Overwhelming workload.

8. Certain essential services (i.e., dietary, housekeeping, professional services) that are identified for private sector contracting may not be available in the immediate area, cost more than federal FTE's, might not get what you expected or paid for, etc. For medical contracts the costs may be shifted to the already overextended CHS budget.

9. Termination of positions result in loss of technical expertise in the organization.

10. Overworked staff and shortage of personnel result in burned out staff, unsafe patient care, and diminishing preventive measures, i.e., deterioration of the physical environment, decaying facilities, etc. Poor appearance of the facility and poor moral

of the staff will affect public perception of Indian Health Services.

11. **Deterioration of team work due to uncertainty about the future.**

12. **Will private contractors be culturally sensitive and aware.**

13. **With private contracting, there is a possibility of conflict in supervisor authority since contract personnel cannot be technically supervised by IHS personnel.**

14. **Contracting of services is a major headache. The federal procurement system is not set-up to meet the demands, needs, and expectations of a health care delivery system. Its set-up to purchase pencils and paper for non-health care organizations.**

15. **Professionalism and quality of work of contractors are concerns. It is extremely time consuming and lengthy, and involves copious documentation to get rid of contractors which are not meeting contractual requirements. And there is no guarantee that another contractor will be available or meet the contractual requirements set by NAIHS.**

16. **RIF'ing is based on seniority and other factors; therefore, some key personnel may be dismissed and their termination might impact administrative functions and patient care services.**

17. **Restructuring departments/programs/services requires lots of paperwork, i.e., re-do position descriptions, reclassification, and if an employee does not fit the new position description, the organization is stuck with the employee (in an old position description) and a new position description that cannot be filled because its tied up.**

18. **Past history in Navajo Area indicates that current IHS employees in professional positions choose not to work under a 638 Self Determination contract.**

19. **Enhanced recruitment and retention problems with FTE reduction due to uncertain career future.**

20. **638 contracts, private sector contracts, and termination or cutting back services may cause fragmentation of services within a Service Unit or NAIHS; and this action might affect JCAHO accreditation and/or the public's perception of IHS.**

Whatever actions are taken in NAIHS relative to FTE reduction should be consistent throughout Navajo, well thought out and planned, and the consumers should be well informed of the decisions and actions prior to implementation. If it becomes necessary to further reduce FTEs beyond the termination of temporary positions and non-essential permanent vacant positions, it would be more feasible to eliminate entire programs/services for the benefit of maintaining staffing for essential programs/services so health care services are not meager. Lets deliver the best care that we can afford through those

programs/services a Service Unit chooses to retain, instead of creating further mediocrity throughout the Indian Health Services.

Further, I strongly believe there is no "FAT" to be cut in Shiprock Service Unit, like the rest of NAIHS. While we go along with the recommendations for a 16% or greater cut in all major line item programs, it is clear that the diverse and comprehensive services that the Indian Health Services (IHS) provides is what makes the IHS unique and what makes it work. There is no other "health care system" in this country that addresses the real health needs of the public as well as the IHS. One need only look at the immunization rates that are the envy of this country, achieved with minimal resources and maximal innovation and effort. What is being cut is a "bare-bones" operation - and a great bargain, the rest of the country should be learning from the IHS how to provide quality care and public health services for less than 20% of the national per capita costs. Part of the answer lies in the people we have working with us: dedicated and hard-working professionals who all go much further than the "extra mile" for our patients. Doctors, nurses, janitors, and secretaries all have opportunities to make more money - sometimes a lot more money - in other settings, but choose to work with us because they want to make a difference. Their reward for this dedication and accomplishment is that we are talking about cutting a portion or all of their jobs.

Any "cuts" in IHS staffing or services must be made up somewhere. If entire programs are to be cut, then I recommend they be replaced with 638 tribal contracts so that services are still available to the people. It is unlikely that any of this can be done quickly, and I have concerns about losing current quality staff, as well as subjecting vital health programs to the whims of politics, but this is better than losing the services altogether, and at some point such transfers may result in more local responsibility for health care.

The most important parts of the new Shiprock Hospital are our patients and the staff who will work there. Without adequate staff, it is a cruel joke on the people of Shiprock to pretend that the new hospital will be a great leap forward. Also, any plans to move health services under tribal control must not disguise cuts or under funding of these services.

Past history indicates that when resources become minimal, community/public health services are the most likely programs to be targeted for reduction; hence, I have grave concerns about those health promotion programs directly funded by the Service Unit. We have made great steps towards including prevention and health promotion within our scope of services. This is the only approach which is likely to have any impact on the health of our people. If we say that health promotion is part of what we are about - "but only when we can afford it and when we have the time..." - then we will never really do it. If we need to redefine our VISION for NAIHS, I strongly support that HP/DP remain a strong priority for our people. Lets look up stream and prevent health problems and promote good health, instead of dealing with the after effects of poor health. HP/DP becomes much more important when resources for clinical health care is becoming limited in the IHS.

The Navajo Nation and other Indian Nations need to be well informed of the consequences of what FTE reduction will have on them as tribes, communities, and individuals.

Last but not least, the US Government is once again reneging on a solemn promise and agreement with sovereign nations. Legal binding agreements that were entered into good faith between our forefathers and the US Government; hence, the justification for the sole existence of the IHS should not be based on need, poverty, or remoteness, but on a promise. Despite this, there is a great health care need, and no real alternative available as to how to meet the needs.

1 **IMPACT STATEMENT**

NO NEW POSITIONS FOR THE NEW NORTHERN NAVAJO MEDICAL CENTER

Using the upgraded Indian Health Services Staffing Methodology, the Navajo Area Indian Health Services requested 515 positions in December 1993 for the new Northern Navajo Medical Center. However, the president's Budget for Fiscal Year 1995 does not show any new positions for the Northern Navajo Medical Center.

No new positions for the Northern Navajo Medical Center would have a devastating effect on the health care delivery system for the Navajo Indians. The following are examples of what it would mean to our people if we do not get additional staffing for our new hospital:

1. A majority of our people have to travel more then two hours on dirt roads to access medical care on the Navajo reservation. If the Northern Navajo Medical Center is not staffed with health care professionals, where would we go for medical treatment and care that is equivalent to President Clinton's Universal Benefits Package for U.S. citizens?

2. Another broken promise by our US Government, our new hospital will simply become a newer, bigger place where nothing has really changed, we will still have to wait even longer hours to see a doctor and not able to see the same doctor because there are no new doctors and nurses with the new hospital.

3. There will be no Ear, Nose and Throat surgery: there is currently only two ENT physicians for all of Navajo. Our young patients who need "ear tubes" for recurrent ear infections, older patients with ruptured eardrums who need repair, and others needing ENT specialty services would benefit greatly from our own ENT doctor. We currently have an ENT doctor interested in working at the new hospital who is also trained in plastic surgery. His skills would be an immense benefit to our many patients with burns and injuries who need reparative services. ENT specialists are in high demand, and if we lose this interested person, we may not be able to recruit another any time soon because doctors are extremely difficult to recruit to the Indian Health Services.

4. There will be no on-site Orthopedic Surgery: our greatest need is operative repair of traumatic bone injuries, as well as non-operative follow-up of these injuries. The high rate of intentional and unintentional injuries among our people has been well documented. Current Orthopedic services at Shiprock include once a month, overcrowded follow-up clinics from Gallup Indian Hospital orthopedic staff - with no operative orthopedics

services on-site.

5. Expanded scope and volume of dental services and optometry services to meet increasing needs of our growing population are planned for the new hospital. Without dental and optometry staff, we will have to limit such services even more as our population grows. Already we have our people line up for hours to obtain dental or optometry appointments. Currently we are not able to offer prosthetic services like dentures and we only provide a limited portion of the population with ongoing "routine" dental care. We will become more and more an "emergencies only" dental and optometry programs. There is no system available for contracting dentistry and optometry services, contracting out these services is not an option for us.

6. Most critical, without new nursing staff in the outpatient department, we will not be able to offer our patients the improvements in continuity of care that have been planned for the new hospital. The majority of our 140,000 outpatient visits currently are non-appointed ("walk-ins") visits through the "treatment room". For our people this means long waiting times in an overcrowded waiting area, to see a different provider every time, talking about sensitive personal issues in a busy room only walled off by a curtain, and little time for attention to "routine" or preventive care. For the new hospital, we have listened carefully to our people's suggestions and complaints, and designed a system where most patients could see their own doctor, in their own doctor's clinic with both same-day and long term appointments. We will not be able to make these improvements to our high volume service area (outpatient care) if we do not have additional nurses and nursing assistants to make it work. Without additional staff, the U.S. Government is setting itself for failure, failure to provide adequate, safe, and respectful health care services to Native Americans.

7. Without additional administrative-support staff, we have to limit clinical services to even less than what we have now. Do we now ask our doctors, nurses, and other direct care providers to do their own clerical work, expedite their own travel orders, process their own payroll, order their own supplies, procure their own patient supplies, clean-up patient rooms, clean-up operating rooms, etc.

8. We planned and constructed for audiology services for our people in the new hospital, but without audiology staff (we have none now) there will be no such care for our people.

9. After much hard work justifying the need, we are

installing a CT scanner in the new hospital. Currently many of our people have to travel many miles for CT scans. Without additional staff in radiology, we will either have to not use the new scanner, or stop performing some other current radiology services in order to staff the scanner, further inconveniencing our patients, and even forcing some very, very sick patients to take the risks of traveling long distance for tests we have the capability (but not the staff) of performing at the new hospital.

10. Currently we have begun to emphasize prevention, both in the clinic and the community. With limited resources and staffing, this will become even more important. Our efforts have focused on adolescent health, school health education, women's health, injury prevention, AIDs prevention, nutrition and exercise, and domestic violence prevention. There will be pressure to cut back on prevention and health promotion efforts as health resources become limited and services are confined to emergency medical care only. Terminating or decreasing health prevention and health promotion efforts will be a great loss to our communities as well as to the patients we serve. We believe that prevention is the only way that we can effectively address growing problems like increasing rates of violent injury and death, epidemic rates of child and partner abuse, doubling of the rates of diabetes-related amputations, increasing numbers of dialysis patients, and increasing rates of heart disease. As we are just beginning to see diabetes among our children. We have re-dedicated ourselves to prevention. Without new staff, we risk losing this commitment and vision to building a healthier Navajo Nation.

11. Last but not least, the US Government is once again reneging on a solemn promise and agreement with sovereign nations. Legal binding agreements that were entered into good faith between our forefathers and the US Government; hence, the justification for the sole existence of the Indian Health Services (and the Northern Navajo Medical Center) should not be based on need, poverty, or remoteness, but on a promise. Despite this, there is a great health care need, and **no real alternative** available to meet the need.

Thank you

02/15/94

NORTHERN NAVAJO MEDICAL CENTER
SHIPROCK, NEW MEXICO
STAFFING COMPARSION
FY 95 RRMNA AND PRESIDENT'S BUDGET

DEPARTMENT POSITIONS	A NAIHS 95 RRMNA	B PRESIDENT'S BUDGET	A – B DEVIATION
HOSPITALS AND CLINICS			
NURSING			
Additional Need	253	0	253
PRIMARY CARE PROVIDERS			
Additional Need	21	0	21
SUPPORT MEDICAL STAFF			
Additional Need	169	0	169
ADMINISTRATION			
Additional Need	43	0	43
TOTAL H AND C	486	0	486
DENTAL			
DENTISTS			
Additional Need	5	0	5
SUPPORT STAFF			
Additional Need	10	0	10
TOTAL DENTAL	15	0	15
MENTAL HEALTH			
PROFESSIONALS STAFF			
Additional Need	3	0	3
SUPPORT STAFF			
Additional Need	1	0	1
TOTAL MENTAL HEALTH	4	0	4
SANITATION			
ENVIRONMENTAL HEALTH			
Additional Need	1	0	1
TOTAL SANITATION	1	0	1
COMMUNITY HEALTH NURSING			
NURSING STAFF			
Additional Need	6	0	6
SUPPORT STAFF			
Additional Need	3	0	3
TOTAL COMMUNITY HEALTH	9	0	9
TOTAL	515	0	515

02/15/94

NORTHERN NAVAJO MEDICAL CENTER
SHIPROCK, NEW MEXICO
STAFFING COMPARSION
FY 95 RRMNA AND PRESIDENT'S BUDGET AND IHS PROPOSED STAFFING

DEPARTMENT POSITIONS	A NAIHS 95 RRMNA	B PRESIDENT'S BUDGET	C 10 MONTH PROPOSED	A – B DEVIATION	A – C DEVIATION
HOSPITALS AND CLINICS					
NURSING					
Additional Need	253	0	44	253	209
PRIMARY CARE PROVIDERS					
Additional Need	21	0	11	21	10
SUPPORT MEDICAL STAFF					
Additional Need	169	0	44	169	125
ADMINISTRATION					
Additional Need	43	0	9	43	34
TOTAL H AND C	486	0	108	486	378
DENTAL					
DENTISTS					
Additional Need	5	0	9	5	–4
SUPPORT STAFF					
Additional Need	10	0	18	10	–8
TOTAL DENTAL	15	0	27	15	–12
MENTAL HEALTH					
PROFESSIONALS STAFF					
Additional Need	3	0	3	3	0
SUPPORT STAFF					
Additional Need	1	0	0	1	1
TOTAL MENTAL HEALTH	4	0	3	4	1
SANITATION					
ENVIRONMENTAL HEALTH					
Additional Need	1	0	0	1	1
TOTAL SANITATION	1	0	0	1	1
COMMUNITY HEALTH NURSING					
NURSING STAFF					
Additional Need	6	0	3	6	3
SUPPORT STAFF					
Additional Need	3	0	1	3	2
TOTAL COMMUNITY HEALTH	9	0	4	9	5
TOTAL	515	0	142	515	373

The Legislature

of the

State of New Mexico

41st Legislature, 2nd Session

LAWS 1994

CHAPTER

HOUSE MEMORIAL 37

Introduced by

REPRESENTATIVE THOMAS E. ATCITTY
REPRESENTATIVE NICK L. SALAZAR
REPRESENTATIVE LEO C. WATCHMAN, JR.
REPRESENTATIVE FRANK E. PAUL
REPRESENTATIVE LYNDA M. MORGAN
REPRESENTATIVE JAMES ROGER MADALENA
REPRESENTATIVE DEBBIE A. RODELLA

GREAT SEAL OF THE STATE OF NEW MEXICO * 1912 *

A MEMORIAL

REQUESTING THE PRESIDENT, THE UNITED STATES CONGRESS, THE UNITED STATES HEALTH AND HUMAN SERVICES DEPARTMENT AND THE INDIAN HEALTH SERVICE TO FULLY STAFF AND FUND THE NEW SHIPROCK HOSPITAL.

WHEREAS, since 1972 the Shiprock community has struggled yet committed itself to the construction and staffing of a new Shiprock hospital to meet the health care needs of the area; and

WHEREAS, after twenty years of effort the Shiprock hospital is now built, but in December 1993 an executive order was issued by President Clinton to all federal agencies telling them to cut staff; and

WHEREAS, the proposed staffing cuts at the Shiprock hospital mean that no new positions will be funded and that cuts of one hundred five positions will occur throughout the Shiprock service unit; and

WHEREAS, these proposed cuts mean fewer doctors, nurses, janitors, clerks, dentists, eye doctors, public health nurses and environmental health nurses and overall it means fewer health services for the forty-five thousand people in the Shiprock service unit;

NOW, THEREFORE, BE IT RESOLVED BY THE HOUSE OF REPRESENTATIVES OF THE STATE OF NEW MEXICO that the president of the United States, the United States congress, the United States department of health and human services and the Indian health service be requested to renounce and oppose the proposed staffing cuts at the Shiprock hospital; and

BE IT FURTHER RESOLVED that by avoiding these staff cuts the people of the Shiprock service area will be able to fulfill their dream of providing full health services to over forty thousand people; and

BE IT FURTHER RESOLVED that copies of this memorial be transmitted to the president, the congress, the secretary of health and human services and the director of the Indian health service.

IGRMA-67-94

Class "C" Resolution
No BIA Action Required.

RESOLUTION OF THE
INTERGOVERNMENTAL RELATIONS COMMITTEE
OF THE NAVAJO NATION COUNCIL

Requesting the 103rd Congress to Fund an Additional 515 Full-Time Employees in the Amount of $23,610,175 For the New Northern Navajo Medical Center, Shiprock, New Mexico, Enabling the New Facility to Provide the Needed Comprehensive Health Care

WHEREAS:

1. Pursuant to 2 N.T.C., Sections 822 (2) and 824 (b) (3), the purpose of the Intergovernmental Relations Committee is to ensure the presence and voice of the Navajo Nation; and is authorized by Navajo Nation Council to review and continually monitor federal programs and activities, assisting in the development of those programs through intergovernmental relationships between the Navajo Nation and such departments; and

2. The United States Government, through the Indian Health Service, is responsible for providing a comprehensive health services delivery system for American Indians and Alaska Natives; and

3. The United States Government is responsible for providing a comprehensive health services delivery system for the Navajo people as provided for in the Navajo Nation Treaty of 1868; and

4. The Navajo Area Indian Health Service (NAIHS) is anxiously awaiting the opening of the Northern Navajo Medical Center in Shiprock, New Mexico (previously named the Shiprock Comprehensive Health Care Facility) with construction over 60% complete and scheduled to open September 1994; and

5. The 1995 budget request submitted by NAIHS, based on the Required Resource Methodology Needs Assessment (RRMNA), requires additional staffing 515 full-time positions to meet the needs of the new Shiprock Facility to provide comprehensive health services; and

6. The FY 1995 preliminary Indian health Service budget proposed funding for only 10 months of the fiscal year for only 142 additional positions to begin operation of the new facility as outlined in the attached Exhibit "A"; this level will under-utilize the new facility and deny Navajos full medical services; and

7. The FY 1995 United States Budget indicates no funds for additional positions for the new Shiprock hospital. The President has mandated that new hospital positions must be obtained from within the current Indian Health Service position ceiling; and

8. By Executive Order, the Indian Health Service has been directed to reduce full-time equivalent (FTE) positions at all offices. For Shiprock, the projected cuts are as many as 105 from their current staffing. The total additional staff need, as submitted by NAIHS, as required by RRMNA and Program of Requirements, was 515 positions, inclusive of all major line item budget categories. The Shiprock Facility should be funded at 100% of the required need (additional 515 full-time positions) for a 12-month period of FY 1995, as shown in the attached Exhibit "B"; and

9. While there is a need to reduce the size of the Federal Government, the Indian Health Service provides direct services to meet needs which will not dissipate. Shiprock Service Unit provides services to over 45,000 people with growing needs due to diabetes, cancer, the rise in injuries and deaths from automobile accidents, to name a few; and

10. The Shiprock Service Unit is relatively under-resourced with clinical resources of only $489 (Congressional allocation plus Medicare and Medicaid) per person per year compared with the national health care expenditures of over 3,760 per capita per year; and

11. The Health and Social Services Committee of the Navajo Nation Council, by Resolution HSSC-MA-37-94, attached hereto as Exhibit "C", recommends funding for an additional 515 full-time employees in the amount of $23,610,175 for the new Northern Navajo Medical Center, Shiprock, New Mexico, which will enable the facility to provide the needed comprehensive health care as intended by Congress.

NOW THEREFORE BE IT RESOLVED THAT:

1. The Intergovernmental Relations Committee of the Navajo Nation Council hereby requests the 103rd Congress of the United States to fund an additional 515 full-time employees in the amount of $23,610,175 for the new Northern Navajo Medical Center, Shiprock, New Mexico, enabling the new facility to provide needed comprehensive health care.

2. The Intergovernmental Relations Committee of the Navajo Nation Council further solicits support of said request by all appropriate programs, agencies and the appropriate committees of Congress, as well as New Mexico, Arizona and Utah Congressional delegations.

CERTIFICATION

I hereby certify that the foregoing resolution was duly considered by the Intergovernmental Relations Committee of the Navajo Nation Council at a duly called meeting at Window Rock (Navajo Nation), Arizona, at which a quorum was present and that same was passed by a vote of 7 in favor, 0 opposed and 0 abstained, this 28th day of March, 1994.

Nelson Gorman Jr.
Chairman
Intergovernmental Relations Committee

Motion: Elmer Milford
Second: David John

EXHIBIT "C"

HSSC-MA-37-94

RESOLUTION OF THE
HEALTH AND SOCIAL SERVICES COMMITTEE
OF THE NAVAJO NATION COUNCIL

Recommending to the Intergovernmental Relations Committee of the Navajo Nation Council to Request the 103rd Congress to Fund an Additional 515 Full-Time Employees in the Amount of $23,610,175 for the New Northern Navajo Medical Center, Shiprock, New Mexico, Enabling New Facility to Provide the Needed Comprehensive Health Care

WHEREAS:

1. Pursuant to 2 N.T.C. Sections 451 and 454 (b)(1), the Health and Social Services Committee is established as a standing committee of the Navajo Nation Council empowered to represent the Navajo Nation in matters relating to health, social services, and environmental health; and

2. Pursuant to 2 N.T.C. Section 454 (b)(3), the Health and Social Services Committee is empowered to coordinate all health and social services related activities of the Navajo Nation and its enterprises, relating to the delivery of health and social services and health and social services planning and prevention; and

3. The Navajo Area Indian Health Service (NAIHS), is anxiously awaiting the opening of the long-awaited Northern Navajo Medical Center (previously named the Shiprock Comprehensive Heath Care Facility) with construction over 60% complete and scheduled to open September 1994; and

4. Using the upgraded Indian Health Service's Staffing Methodology the Navajo Area Indian Health Service requested 515 positions in December 1993 for the new Northern Navajo Medical Center; however, President Clinton's Budget for Fiscal Year 1995 does not show any new positions for the Northern Navajo Medical Center; and

5. No new positions for the Northern Navajo Medical Center would have a devastating effect on the health care delivery systems for the Navajo Indians. Examples, longer waiting time, exceeding 3 to 4 hours; no additional doctors and nurses will compound the existing manpower shortage; the immunization level falling below 95%; the infant mortality rate dropping below the national average; termination of several inpatient services and public health services; sending the Navajo people off the reservation to hospitals that are culturally insensitive; nor speak the language of the Navajo people; cessation of the much needed health promotion and disease prevention activities, etc. see impact statement attached as Exhibit "A"; and

HSSC-MA-37-94

6. The Shiprock Service Unit is relatively under-resource with clinical resources of only $489 (Congressional allocation plus Medicare and Medicaid) per person per year compared with the national health care expenditures of over $3,760 per capita per year.

NOW THEREFORE BE IT RESOLVED THAT:

1. The Health and Social Services Committee of the Navajo Nation Council recommends to the Intergovernmental Relations Committee of the Navajo Nation Council to request the 103rd Congress to fund an additional Navajo Medical Center, Shiprock, New Mexico enabling the new facility to provide needed comprehensive health care as intended by Congress.

2. The Health and Social Services Committee of the Navajo Nation Council further recommends the Navajo Area Indian Health Service place the staffing for the new Shiprock Hospital a top priority of the Navajo Area Indian Health Service for FY 1995 and, thereafter, the staffing be a recurring budget item in the Indian Health Service Budget.

CERTIFICATION

I hereby certify that the foregoing resolution was duly considered by the Health and Social Services Committee at a duly called meeting at Window Rock, Navajo Nation (Arizona), at which a quorum was present and that same was passed by a vote of 5 in favor, 0 opposed, and 0 opposed, this 25th day of March, 1994.

Vice Chairman
Health and Social Services Committee

Motioned by: John Gould
Seconded by: Martin Bahe

Dzilth-na-o-dith-hle Health Advisory Board
Dzilth-na-o-dith-hle Health Center
Star Route 4, Box 5400
Bloomfield, New Mexico 87413

RESOLUTION OF THE DZILTH-NA-O-DITH-HLE HEALTH ADVISORY BOARD
DZHB-94-001

SUBJECT: Opposing the Clinton Administration Across-the-Board Staff Reduction and Requesting a Waiver for Federal Health Care Provider Organizations, such as the Indian Health Service.

WHEREAS:

1. The Dzilth-na-o-dith-hle Health Center Advisory Board was established with approval of the Tribal Chapters (Huerfano, Nageezi, Counselors), Shiprock Service Unit Health Board (11-25-86), and the Navajo Area Indian Health Service Health Board (03-23-87), and;

2. The five member committee was appointed by respective chapters at duly called meetings, and;

3. The Dzilth-na-o-dith-hle Health Center Health Advisory Board, by approved by-laws, represents the interest of the Indian people receiving health care in this service area, and;

4. The Dzilth-na-o-dith-hle Health Center Health Advisory Board serves in an official advisory capacity to the Dzilth-na-o-dith-hle Health Center Director regarding all health, health related plans and operations, and;

5. The Dzilth-na-o-dith-hle Health Center Health Advisory Board initiates goals, objectives and plans in cooperation with the Health Center Director and the Navajo Area Indian Health Service Director.

THEREFORE BE IT RESOLVED THAT:

1. The Dzilth-na-o-dith-hle Health Board is opposing the proposed FTE reductions and requests a waiver for federal health care provider organization, such as the Indian Health Service.

2. The Dzilth-na-o-dith-hle Health Advisory Board is opposing any staff reduction plans involving direct patient care facilities.

3. The Dzilth-na-o-dith-hle Health Advisory Board is requesting the Navajo Indian Health Service to de-centraling support/financial services to the local facilities to provide an efficient support services.

CERTIFICATION

We hereby certify that the foregoing resolution was duly presented and discussed at a duly called meeting of the Dzilth-na-o-dith-hle Health Center Health Advisory Board, motioned by Lee Norberto, seconded by Lula Hacessa. Passed with a vote of 5 in favor, and 0 opposed, this 10th day of 1994.

Ervin Chavez
President

HOGBACK COMMUNITY CHAPTER

RESOLUTION OF THE HOGBACK COMMUNITY CHAPTER
HOGB-9401-04

REQUESTING THE U.S. CONGRESS TO ADD $9.2 MILLION TO THE FY. 1995 INDIAN HEALTH SERVICE BUDGET FOR THE ADDITIONAL 264 FULL-TIME POSITIONS TO FULL STAFF THE NORTHERN NAVAJO MEDICAL CENTER IN SHIPROCK, NEW MEXICO.

WHEREAS:

1. *The Hogback Chapter is a legally certified Navajo Nation Chapter, pursuant to Navajo Tribal Council Resolution CAP 36-78, and thus has the authority to make appropriate recommendations to the Navajo Nation, or such Federal, State, County, and Navajo Nation agencies for review and enactment on matter of local community concerns; And,*

2. *The communities of the Northern Navajo Nation are anxiously awaiting the opening of the Northern Navajo Medical Center. The Northern Navajo Medical Center construction is costing the United States citizens more than $50 million. The construction is more than 70% complete and the new facility is scheduled to put into operation in early September 1994; And,*

3. *The IHS staffing methodology had identified and justified 264 additional positions to meet the staffing needs of the new Northern Navajo Medical Center to provide comprehensive medical services as intended by the U.S. Congress; And,*

4. *U.S. President Bill Clinton's FY 1995 budget does not include funding for additional positions in the new Northern Navajo Medical Center. The staff increases must be offset with contracts for services but no additional resources is proposed to offset the imminent additional contracting costs; And,*

5. *The current staffing at the Shiprock PHS/IHS Indian Hospital is already inadequate to fully utilize the new medical center. The level of services provided at the old hospital will be duplicated at the new facility due to lack of additional staff.*

NOW THEREFORE BE IT RESOLVED THAT:

1. *The Hogback Chapter hereby respectfully requests the U.S. Congress to appropriate additional $9.2 million to the FY 1995 IHS budget for the additional 264 full-time positions to fully meet the required staffing for the Northern Navajo Medical Center, Shiprock, New Mexico.*

2. Further, the Hogback Chapter respectfully requests the U.S. Congress to coordinate strategies to increase the Indian Health Care funds to remedy the already underfunded Indian Health Services budget.

C E R T I F I C A T I O N

We hereby certify that the foregoing resolution was considered by the Hogback Chapter at a duly called chapter meeting at Hogback, NM at which a quorum was present. **Davidson DeVore** *made a motion and* **Daisy Johnson** *seconded the motion. The same was passed with 28 in favor, 0 opposed, and 0 abstained this 23rd day of January 1994.*

Jimmy Woody,
Chapter President

Paul George,
Chapter Vice-President

Eddie K. Etcitty
Chapter Secretary/Treasurer

George Kellywood, Sr.
Council Delegate

xc: Chapter Government, Shiprock Agency
: Chapter File

FEB 1994
Received
Community Services
Development Department
Shiprock Agency

Naakaii To'

Mexican Water Chapter

HCR 6100 Box 38-618
Teec Nos Pos, AZ 86514
(602) 674-3641

David L. John, Council Delegate
Marlin Saggboy, Chapter President
Francis Haskan Sr., Chapter Vice President
Secretary / Treasurer
Luke G. Sagg, Grazing Representative
Community Services Coordina

**PROPOSED RESOLUTION OF THE
MEXICAN WATER CHAPTER**

REQUESTING THE UNITED STATES CONGRESS TO ADD $9.2 MILLION TO THE FISCAL YEAR 1995 INDIAN HEALTH SERVICE BUDGET FOR AN ADDITIONAL 264 FULL-TIME EMPLOYEES TO STAFF THE NORTHERN NAVAJO MEDICAL CENTER, SHIPROCK, NEW MEXICO:

WHEREAS:

1. The Mexican Water Community Chapter was certified by the Navajo Tribal Council per Resolution CAP-32-78 and thus has the authority to make appropriate recommendations to the Navajo Nation, or such Federal, State, County, and Tribal agencies for review and enactment on matters of local concern; and

2. The communities of the northern Navajo reservation are anxiously awaiting the opening of the Northern Navajo Medical Center (previously named the Shiprock Comprehensive Health Care Facility). The construction is 60% complete and the new facility is scheduled to open in September, 1994; and

3. The Indian Health Services staffing methodology identified and justified 264 additional positions to meet the staffing needs of the new Shiprock facility and provide comprehensive medical services as intended by congress; and

4. President Clinton's Fiscal Year 1995 budget indicates no funds for additional positions for the new Shiprock Hospital. The staff increases must be offset with contracts for services, but no additional resources is proposed to offset the imminent additional contracting costs; and

5. The current staffing is inadequate to fully utilize the new hospital. Lack of additional staff will result in the level of services currently provided at the old hospital remaining the same in the new facility.

NOW THEREFORE BE IT RESOLVED THAT:

1. The Mexican Water Chapter hereby respectfully requests the United States Congress to add $9.2 million to the Fiscal Year 1995 Indian Health Services budget for an additional 264 full-time employee to staff the Northern Navajo Medical Center, Shiprock, New Mexico.

Page Two (02)
Chapter Resolution
S/R Sterring Committee

C E R T I F I C A T I O N

We, hereby certify that the foregoing resolution was fully discussed and considered at a duly called Chapter Meeting at (Mexican Water, Navajo Nation, Arizona), at which a quorum was present and that same was approved and passed by a vote of 28 infavor; 0 opposed, and 5 abstained this 13th day of February, 1994.

C O N C U R R E N C E :

David L. John, Council Delegate

Marlin Saggboy, Chapter President

Francis Haskan Sr., Vice President

(Pro Temp) Secretary

Resolution of the Red Valley Chapter RV-94-98

Navajo Nation, Red Valley, Arizona

IN SUPPORT OF FULLY STAFFING THE NEW SHIPROCK PHS HOSPITAL TO MEET THE HEALTH NEEDS OF THE SHIPROCK AREA, AND IN OPPOSITION TO PLANS TO CUTBACK ON CURRENT STAFFING LEVELS.

WHEREAS:

1. The Red Valley Chapter was established and certified pursuant to Resolution CMY-023-79, by the Navajo Tribal Council and gave it certain authorities to enact pertaining to the local community; and

2. The Shiprock Service Unit of the Navajo Area Indian Health Service is charged with providing health service to over 45,000 residents of the Northern Navajo area: and

3. In 1972 the United States Congress recognized the need for a new hospital in the Northern Navajo area and appropriated over $1 million dollars for the design of a new hospital, but no funds were appropriated for the construction of the hospital; and

4. Over the subsequent 21 years, community members repeatly requested expanded staff and services to meet the needs of a growing population, but were informed that the only way to get a significant increase in health resources was to be approved for a new facility; and

5. The Navajo Nation, the Shiprock Hospital Steering Committee, and the 21 chapters of the Shiprock Service Unit worked diligently for many years to have a new facility approved, designed, and constructed; and

6. The United States Congress affirmed the need for additional resources by approving and appropriating funds for the construction of the Northern Navajo Medical Center in Shiprock, construction of this facility is scheduled for completion in late 1994; and

7. The Indian Health Service planning methodolgy indicates a need for 264 additional staff positions to meet the health care needs of the people of the Northern Navajo area; and

8. The Indian Health Service plans for FY' 1995 call for no new positions for the Shiprock Hospital and in fact, current federal directives calls for cuts of approximately 100 positions form the present Shiprock service Unit staff; and

9. This will result in the increased use of contracts for health services which will cause loss of local experienced staff, higher costs, and there are increased resources provided for in the FY' 1995 IHS Budget to pay for such contracts; and

10. Whereas, implementation of these plans will result in significant limitations in services to the people.

NOW, THEREFORE BE IT RESOLVED THAT:

1. The Shiprock Planning Commission supports fully funding the 264 additional positions identified as needed for the new Shiprock hospital; and

2. The Shiprock Planning Commission strongly and unequivocally opposes any plans to cut back on current staffing; and

3. The Shiprock Planning Commission calls on the leaders of the Navajo Nation, congressional representatives, and the staff of the Indian Health Service to work to make sure that health care resources available to our people are adequate to meet their needs, and comparable to resources available nationaly; and

4. The Shiprock Planning Commission calls on the Executive branch of the federal government and the United States Congress to honor its treaty obligation to provide for the health care needs of the Navajo people.

C-E-R-T-I-F-I-C-A-T-I-O-N

We the undersigned, certify that the above resolution was presented and thoroughly discussed at a duly called meeting, at which a quorum was present, and the same was approved by a vote of 37 in favor and 0 opposed with 3 abstention on this 23rd day of January, 1994.

Lee B. Roy, Council Delegate

George Tutt, Chapter President

Phillip Harrison, Chapter Vice-President

Rose Chavez, Chapter Secretary

ROCK POINT CHAPTER

BOX 190
ROCK POINT, ARIZONA 86545
(602) 659–4211
(602) 659–4236
FAX (602) 659–4271

NAVAJO NATION COUNCIL
JOHNNY DESCHENY, Council Delegate

CHAPTER OFFICIALS
MITCHELL BURNS, President
WALLACE J. BEGAY, Vice-President
NANCY J. HARVEY, Secretary-Treasurer

RPC-94-016

RESOLUTION OF THE ROCK POINT CHAPTER

REQUESTING THE U.S. CONGRESS TO ADD $9.2 MILLION TO THE FY 1995 IHS BUDGET FOR AN ADDITIONAL 264 FULL-TIME EMPLOYEES TO STAFF THE NORTHERN NAVAJO MEDICAL CENTER, SHIPROCK, NEW MEXICO.

WHEREAS:

1. The Rock Point Community Chapter was certified by the Navajo Tribal Council per Resolution CJ-20-55 and thus has the authority to make appropriate recommendations to the Navajo Nation, or such Federal, State, County, and Tribal agencies for review and enactment on matters of local concern; and

2. The communities of the northern Navajo reservation are anxiously awaiting the opening of the Northern Navajo Medical Center (previously named the Shiprock Comprehensive Health Care Facility). The construction is 60% complete and the new facility is scheduled to open in September 1994; and

3. The IHS staffing methodology identified and justified 264 additional positions to meet the staffing needs of the new Shiprock facility and provide comprehensive medical services as intended by Congress; and

4. President Clinton's FY 1995 budget indicates no funds for additional positions for the new Shiprock Hospital. The staff increases must be offset with contracts for services, but no additional resources is proposed to offset the imminent additional contracting costs; and

5. The current staffing is inadequate to fully utilize the new hospital. Lack of additional staff will result in the level of services currently provided at the old hospital remaining the same in the new facility.

NOW THEREFORE BE IT RESOLVED THAT:

1. The Rock Point Chapter hereby respectfully requests the U.S. Congress to add $9.2 million to the FY 1995 IHS budget for an additional 264 full time employees to staff the Northern Navajo Medical Center, Shiprock, New Mexico.

HARRISON W. BEGAY, Community Services Coordinator • CHARLENE LEE, Clerk-Typist • JAMES W. BEGAY, Grazing Commit

78-786 - 94 - 4

CERTIFICATION

WE HEREBY CERTIFY THAT THE FOREGOING RESOLUTION WAS DULY CONSIDERED BY THE ROCK POINT CHAPTER AT A DULY CALLED MEETING AT ROCK POINT NAVAJO NATION (ARIZONA), AT WHICH A QUORUM WAS PRESENT AND THAT SAME WAS PASSED BY A VOTE OF 59 IN FAVOR AND 0 OPPOSED, THIS 6th DAY OF February, 1994.

CONCURRENCE:

Mitchell Burns
MITCHELL BURNS, CHAPTER PRESIDENT

Wallace J. Begay
WALLACE J. BEGAY, CHAPTER VICE-PRESIDENT

Nancy J. Harvey
NANCY J. HARVEY, CHAPTER SECRETARY/
TREASURE

Johnny Descheny
JOHNNY DESCHENY, COUNCIL DELEGATE

1ST MOTION: Lucy R. Jones

2ND MOTION: Nellie T. John

SANJ-94-064

SAN JUAN CHAPTER

RESOLUTION OF THE SAN JUAN CHAPTER

REQUESTING THE INDIAN HEALTH SERVICES TO INCLUDE FUNDS INTO ITS BUDGET OF $23,610,175 FOR ADDITIONAL 515 POSITIONS FOR THE NORTHERN NAVAJO MEDICAL CENTER, SHIPROCK, NEW MEXICO.

WHEREAS:

1. Pursuant to Resolution #CD-86-81 of the Navajo Tribal Council, the San Juan Chapter has been certified as a recognized body of the Navajo Nation and authorized to conduct business of the local government; and

2. The replacement of the Shiprock Indian Hospital has been in the plans for many years. The project finally commenced in 1987 when Congress appropriated the design funds. Construction funds was appropriated subsequently and construction will be completed on August 1, 1994; and

3. Using the upgraded Indian Health Services Staffing Methodology, the Navajo Area Indian Health Services requested 515 positions in December 1993 for the new Northern Navajo Medical Center. However, the President's Budget for Fiscal Year 1995 does not show any new positions for the Northern Navajo Medical Center; and

4. No new positions for the Northern Navajo Medical Center would have a devastating effect on the health care delivery system for the Navajo Indians. Examples, longer waiting time, exceeding 3 to 4 hours; no doctors and nurses will compound the existing manpower shortage; our immunization level falling below 95%; our infant mortality rate dropping below the national average; termination of several inpatient services and public health services; sending our people off the reservation to hospitals that are not culturally sensitive, nor speak the language of our people; cessation of the much needed health promotion and disease prevention activities, etc; and

5. A majority of our people have to travel more than 2 hours on dirt roads to access any medical care on the Navajo reservation. The new Northern Navajo Medical Center is the only Indian Health Hospital available to the Indian people of Northern Navajo.

NOW, THEREFORE BE IT RESOLVED THAT:

1. The San Juan Chapter hereby requests the Indian Health Services to include funds into its budget of $23,610,175 for additional 515 positions for the Northern Navajo Medical Center, Shiprock, New Mexico.

George Arthur, *Council Delegate* • Stanley Benally, *President* • Wilbert C. Begay, *Vice President* • Shirley Yazzie, *Secretary/Treasurer* • Jerome Bena..., *Grazing Member*

P. O. Box 417 • Waterflow, New Mexico 87421 • (505) 598-6916 • Fax: (505) 598-0021

We hereby certify that the foregoing resolution was duly considered by the San Juan Chapter at a duly called meeting at San Juan Chapter, New Mexico, at which a quorum was present and that the same was passed by a vote of 25 in favor and 0 opposed, and 0 abstained, this 21st day of February, 1994.

George Arthur, Council Delegate

Stanley Benally, President

Wilbert C. Begay, Vice-President

Shirley Yazzie, Secretary/Treasurer

Sheep Springs Chapter

P.O. Drawer "I" • Sheep Springs, NM 87364 • District 12
(505) 732-4288

RESOLUTION

ADOPTING AND APPROVING THE OPPOSITION OF CUTS IN THE INDIAN HEALTH SERVICE STAFFING AND PROGRAMS ON THE NAVAJO NATION AND INDIAN COUNTRY

WHEREAS:

1. The Sheep Springs Chapter, under the authority of the Navajo Nation Tribal Council, is a sovereign and recognized Chapter entity under the Navajo Nation Tribal Government, whose primary purpose is to protect the health, safety and welfare of the Navajo people within it's jurisdiction; and,

2. Policy direction and administrative decisions regarding restructuring of the Federal Government by President Clinton's administration has created uncertainty and instability in the direct health care services to the Navajo people and other Indian Tribes; and,

3. The Sheep Springs Chapter is a strong advocate of the following:
   a) Indian Health Care is a treaty obligation of the United States Government.
   b) Indian Health Service is the designated primary health Care provider of the Navajo people and other Indian Tribes.
   Health Care should not be diminished, for sovereign tribal entities and native communities, due to stipulations under the umbrella of treaty obligations; and

4. The Sheep Springs Chapter is in total opposition to the following:
   a) Any cuts in the 1994-5 budget affecting the delivery of health care to the Navajo people.
   b) The projected 1994-5 reduction in staffing of Indian Health Service in administration and direct service personnel that adversely affects the health care of the Navajo people.
   c) Relocation of the Navajo Area Indian Health Service away from the Navajo Nation property.
   d) Any further planning or actions regarding restructuring by the Clinton Administration regarding Indian Health Service without consultation with the Navajo Nation and other Indian Tribes.

NOW THEREFORE BE IT RESOLVED:

1. The Sheep Springs Chapter recommends that the Navajo Nation Council take the following actions to insure the Clinton Administration protects the health and welfare of the Navajo people and the Indian Tribes by supporting the Indian Health Service:

   a) Waive/exempt all planned staffing cuts.
   b) Waive/exempt all planned budget cuts.
   c) Equity and parity funding of Indian Health Service to the level of non-Indian health care facilities.

d) Funding level at $6.335 billion over the next five years to allow Indian Health Service to provide comprehensive health benefits.

e) Meeting be held with the President and his key management staff on Health Care to include:
   1. First Lady Hillary Rodham Clinton
   2. Donna Shalala
   3. Philip Lee
   4. Leon Panetta
   5. John Hart
   6. Loretta Avante
   7. Greg Stepanoupoulus

f) Meetings with Senate and Congressional committees having jurisdiction over Indian Health Care.

2. The Sheep Springs Chapter recommends the Navajo Nation and other Indian Tribes direct President Clinton and the U.S. Government to adhere to the Federal Indian Policy of continous tribal consultation with elected tribal officials and Tribal sovereign governments in decisions regarding Indian policy and the affects on Indian people. That the Indian Health Service be allowed to improve the delivery of quality health care to its Native American clients without fear of budget cuts and staff reduction.

CERTIFICATION

We, hereby, certify that the foregoing resolution was dicussed, considered and thus supported by Sheep Springs Chapter at a duly called meeting at Sheep Springs, Navajo Nation, New Mexico, at which a quorum was present and that same was passed by a vote of 31 in favor, and 0 opposed, on this 13th day of February 94.

Leonard H. Sandman

Leonard H. Sandman, President

Kenneth Denetclaw Sr.

Kennth Denetclaw Sr., Vice-President

Edison Wood

Edison Woods, Sec/Treas.

John A. Gould Sr.

John A. Gould Sr., Council Delegate

Resolution of the _____Sheep Springs_____ Chapter

REQUESTING THE INDIAN HEALTH SERVICES TO INCLUDE FUNDS INTO ITS BUDGET OF $23,610,175 FOR ADDITIONAL 515 POSITIONS FOR THE NORTHERN NAVAJO MEDICAL CENTER, SHIPROCK, NEW MEXICO

REQUESTING THE U.S. CONGRESS TO INCLUDE INTO THE FISCAL YEAR 1995 FEDERAL BUDGET ADD-ON FUNDS OF $23,610,175 FOR ADDITIONAL 515 POSITIONS FOR THE NORTHERN NAVAJO MEDICAL CENTER, SHIPROCK, NEW MEXICO

WHEREAS:

1. Pursuant to Resolution __________ of the Navajo Tribal Council, the _____Sheep Springs_____ Chapter has been certified as a recognized body of the Navajo Nation and authorized to conduct business of the local government; and

2. The replacement of the Shiprock Indian Hospital has been in the plans for many years. The project finally commenced in 1987 when Congress appropriated the design funds. Construction funds was appropriated subsequently and construction will be completed on August 1, 1994; and

3. Using the upgraded Indian Health Services Staffing Methodology, the Navajo Area Indian Health Services requested 515 positions in December 1993 for the new Northern Navajo Medical Center. However, the President's Budget for Fiscal Year 1995 does not show any new positions for the Northern Navajo Medical Center; and

4. No new positions for the Northern Navajo Medical Center would have a devastating effect on the health care delivery system for the Navajo Indians. Examples, longer waiting time, exceeding 3 to 4 hours; no doctors and nurses will compound the existing manpower shortage; our immunization level falling below 95%; our infant mortality rate dropping below the national average; termination of several inpatient services and public health services; sending our people off the reservation to hospitals that are not culturally sensitive, nor speak the language of our people; cessation of the much needed health promotion and disease prevention activities, etc; and

5. A majority of our people have to travel more than 2 hours on dirt roads to access any medical care on the Navajo reservation. The new Northern Navajo Medical Center is the only Indian Health Hospital available to the Indian people of Northern Navajo.

NOW, THEREFORE BE IT RESOLVED THAT:

1. The Sheep Springs Chapter hereby request the Indian Health Services to include funds into its budget of $23,610,175 for additional 515 positions for the Northern Navajo Medical Center, Shiprock, New Mexico.

2. The Sheep Springs Chapter hereby request of the U.S. Congress to include into the Fiscal Year 1995 Federal Budget add-on funds of $23,610,175 for additional 515 positions for the Northern Navajo Medical Center, Shiprock, New Mexico.

C E R T I F I C A T I O N

We, hereby certify that the foregoing resolution was duly considered by the Sheep Springs Chapter at a duly called meeting at Shiprock, New Mexico, at which a quorum was present and that the same was passed by a vote of 31 in favor and 0 opposed, and 0 abstained, this 13th of February '94 1994.

Leonard Sandoman
President

Kenneth Benaldaw Sr.
Vice President

Edison Wood
Secretary

Council Delegate

Council Delegate

Council Delegate

NAVAJO NATION

RESOLUTION OF THE SHIPROCK CHAPTER

94-01-0024-SHIP

CHAPTER OFFICERS
William Lee
President
David C. Curley
Vice President
Lula Jackson
Secretary / Treasurer

TRIBAL COUNCIL DELEGATES
Wallace Charley
Genevieve Jackson
William Tso
Duane "Chili" Yazzie

AGRICULTURE OFFICERS
David Burbank
Grazing Committee
Robert Hayes
Landboard Member

REQUESTING THE 103rd CONGRESS TO FUND AN ADDITIONAL 264 FULL TIME EMPLOYEES IN THE AMOUNT OF $9.2 MILLION FOR THE NEW NORTHERN NAVAJO MEDICAL CENTER, SHIPROCK, NEW MEXICO. ENABLING THE NEW FACILITY TO PROVIDE THE NEEDED COMPREHENSIVE HEALTH CARE.

WHEREAS:

1. The Shiprock Chapter persuant to the authority contained in Section 1, Subsection (c) of Tribal Council Resolution #W-20-55 which certified Shiprock Chapter as a recognized of the N.N. and is authorized to conduct business of the local goverment, and

2. The United States Government, through the Indian Health Service, is responsible for providing a comprehensive health services delivery system for American Indians and Alaska Natives; and

3. The United States Government is responsible for providing a comprehensive health services delivery system for the Navajo people as provided for in the Navajo Nation Treaty of 1868; and

4. The Shiprock Community people are anxiously awaiting the opening of the Northern Navajo Medical Center (previously named the Shiprock Comprehensive Healthcare Facility) with construction over 60% complete and scheduled to open September 1994; and

5. The 1995 Budget request submitted by NAIHS, based on the Required Resource Methodology Needs Assessment (RRMNA), requires additional staffing of 264 full-time positions to meet the needs of the new Shiprock Facility to provide comprehensive services; and

6. The FY 1995 preliminary IHS budget proposed funding for only 10 months of the fiscal year for only 142 additional positions to begin operation of the new facility as outlined in the attached Exhibit "A"; this level will under utilize the new facility and den Navajos full medical services; and

RESOLUTION OF THE
SHIPROCK CHAPTER
RESOL. NO. 94-01-0024-SHIP
PAGE 02 OF 02

7. The FY 1995 United States Budget indicates no funds for additional positions for the new Shiprock hospital. The president has mandated that new hospital positions must be obtained from within the current IHS position ceiling; and

8. By Executive Order, the Indian Health Service has been directed to reduce full-time equivalent (FTE) positions at all offices. For Shiprock, the projected cuts are as many as 105 from their current staffing. the total additional staff need as submitted by NAIHS as required by RRMNA and Program of Requirements was 264 full-time positions, inclusive of all Major Line Item Budget categories. The Shiprock facility should be funded at 100% of the required need (additional 264 full-time positions) for a 12-month period in FY 1995 as shown in the attached Exhibit "B: and

9. While there is a need to reduce the size of the federal government, the Indian Health Service provides direct services to meet needs which will not disappear. Shiprock Service Unit provides services to over 45,000 people, with growing needs due to diabetes, cancer; the rise in injuries and deaths from automobile accidents, to name a few; and

10. The Shiprock Service Unit is relatively under-resourced with a Congressional allocation of only $333 per persons per year compared with the national health care expenditures of over $3,000 per capital per year; and

11. The Shiprock Chapter by Resolution recommends funding for an additional 264 full-time employees in the amount of $9.2 million for the New Northern Navajo Medical Center, Shiprock, New Mexico which will enable the facility to provide the needed comprehensive health care as intended by Congress.

NOW, THEREFORE BE IT RESOLVED THAT§

1. The Shiprock Chapter hereby requests the 103rd Congress of the United States to fund an additional 264 full-time employees in the amount of $9.2 million for the New Northern Navajo Medical Center, Shiprock, New Mexico, enabling the new facility to provide needed comprehensive health care.

2. The Shiprock Chapter further solicits supports of said request by all appropriate programs, agencies and the appropriate committees of Congress, and New Mexico, Arizona Congressional Delegations.

RESOLUTION OF THE
SHIPROCK CHAPTER
RESOL. NO. 94-01-0024-SHIP
PAGE 03 OF 03

C E R T I F I C A T I O N

I hereby certify that the foregoing resolutions was duty considered by the Navajo Nation Council at a duly called meeting at Window Rock, Navajo Nation (Arizona), at which a quorum was present and that same was passed by a vote of 62 in favor 00 opposed and 00 abstained this 23 day of January 1994.

WILLIAM LEE,
President

DUANE H. YAZZIE,
Council Delegate

DAVID C. CURLEY
Vice President

WILLIAM TSO,
Council Delegate

LULA JACKSON
Sec./Treasurer

GENEVIEVE JACKSON
Council Delegate

WALLACE CHARLEY
Council Delegate

TWO GREY HILLS CHAPTER

Cornelia M. Shorty
President

James Hunt, Sr.
Vice-President

Albert Lee
Secretary / Treasurer

Frankie Hunt
Grazing Member

Richard Begay
Council Delegate

"Home of the famous Two Grey Hills Rugs"

RESOLUTION

TGH 94-03-13-01

REQUESTING THE INDIAN HEALTH SERVICES TO INCLUDE FUNDS INTO ITS BUDGET OF $23,610,175 FOR ADDITIONAL 515 POSITIONS FOR THE NORTHERN NAVAJO MEDICAL CENTER, SHIPROCK, NEW MEXICO

WHEREAS:

1. The Two Grey Hills Chapter is a certified body of Government for the communities of Toadlena, Two Grey Hills, Blackhouse Valley and South Tocito; AND

2. The replacement of the Shiprock Indian Hospital has been in the plans for many years. The project finally commenced in 1987 when Congress appropriated the design funds. Construction funds was appropriated subsequently and construction will be completed on August 1, 1994; AND

3. Using the upgraded Indian Health Services Staffing Methodology, the Navajo Area Indian Health Service requested 515 positions in December 1993 for the new Northern Navajo Medical Center. However, the President's Budget for Fiscal Year 1995 does not show any new positions for the Northern Navajo Medical Center; AND

4. No new positions for the Northern Navajo Medical Center would have a devastating effect on the health care delivery system for the Navajo Indians. Examples, longer waiting time, exceeding 3 to 4 hours; no doctors and nurses will compound the existing manpower shortage; our immunization level falling below 95%; our infant mortality rate dropping below the national average; termination of several inpatient services and public health services; sending our people off the reservation to hospitals that are not culturally sensitive, nor speak the language of our people; cessation of the much needed health promotion and disease prevention activities, etc; AND

5. A majority of our people have to travel more than 2 hours on dirt roads to access any medical care on the Navajo reservation. The new Northern Navajo Medical Center is the only Indian Health Hospital available to the Indian people of Northern Navajo.

NOW, THEREFORE BE IT RESOLVED THAT:

1. The Two Grey Hills Chapter hereby request the Indian Health Services to include funds into its budget of $23,610,175 for additional 515 positions for the Northern Navajo Medical Center, Shiprock, New Mexico.

C E R T I F I C A T I O N

We, hereby, certify that the foregoing resolution was duly considered by the Two Grey Hills, Navajo Nation, New Mexico at which a quorum was present and that same was passed by a vote of 41 in favor and 0 opposed, this 13th day of March, 1994.

Cornelia Shorty, President

James Hunt, Vice-President

Albert Lee, Sec./Treasurer

Richard Begay, Council Delegate

P. O. Box 7950 • Newcomb, N.M. 87455 • (505) 789-3232 • FAX (505) 789-3232

VOL. XXXIIII NO. 02 • Thursday, January 13, 1994

No money, no sense

By BILL DONOVAN
Navajo Times Correspondent

SHIPROCK - The new $45 million Shiprock Indian Health Service Hospital will open to a lot of empty corridors next fall, unless someone is able to find the money to hire new personnel.

That was the word Tuesday from U.S. Sen. Pete Domenici, IHS personnel and Navajo officials.

Domenici met for about half an hour with Navajo President Peterson Zah and one of the subjects that came under discussion was what to do about the Shiprock Hospital situation.

The opening of the new hospital couldn't come at a worst time... Although money was provided for building the hospital and purchasing new equipment, IHS officials said no money was provided for new personnel.

So, what is going to happen, said Genevieve Jackson, one of Shiprock's council delegates, is that "the old staff from the old hospital will be transferred over there. No new personnel will be hired."

In fact, if the reduction in staff goes through as expected, some 50 or so of the staff at the present Shiprock facility may not be going over to the new facility and that means the new facility will have even less personnel than the current hospital, she said.

Duane Beyal, press aide to Zah, said the whole situation doesn't make sense.

"Why spend the tens of millions of dollars to build a new hospital and provide only enough staff to use half of it. All that's going to happen is that you will have the same understaffed and overcrowded conditions at the new facility," he said.

Domenici said he also doesn't think it makes much sense and promised tribal officials that he would support their efforts to get funds to hire enough personnel to fully open the new facility.

Beyal said that because of the good weather, the IHS has told the tribe that the scheduled opening this December has been pushed up to August.

VOL. XXXIIII NO. 05 • Thursday, FEBRUARY 3, 1994

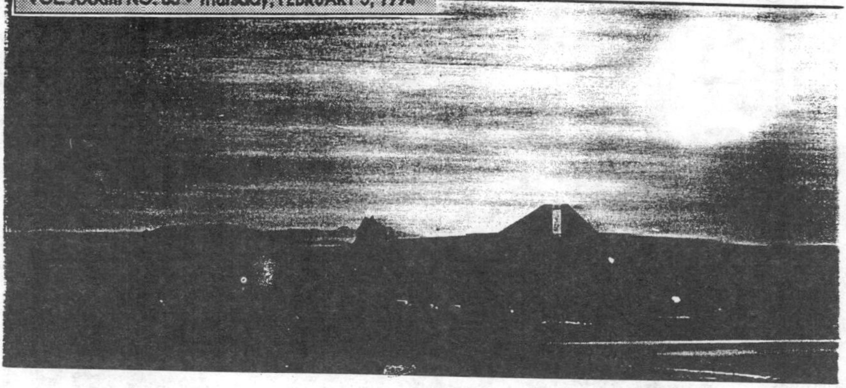

Twin Towers

The new Shiprock Indian Health Service hospital appears to have wings of its own as it stands silhouetted against the 'The Rock with Wings' (Shiprock) in the background, is well ahead of its completion date of September 1994. (Times phc Paul Natonabah)

Zah seeks meeting with Clinto

Hopes to voice objections on proposed cuts

WINDOW ROCK - Navajo Nation President Peterson Zah is lobbying this week in Washington, D.C. against proposed cuts in the Indian Health Service and will have meetings in the White House with Clinton Administration officials.

Zah is also seeking a meeting with President Bill Clinton or First Lady Hillary Rodham Clinton.

On Wednesday, Zah met with Ira Magaziner, Senior Advisor to President Clinton on Policy Development, who is the chief White House aide for health reform.

Zah will be lobbying against the proposed cuts which would eliminate 500 to 600 jobs in the Navajo Area Indian Health Service.

"At a time when Indian people are already under-served and health care on Indian reservations is under-funded, it is inconceivable that Indian health would be forced to take even more cuts," Zah said.

A special case for the Navajo Nation is the staffing of the new Shiprock Hospital which, under the proposed cuts, would receive only 142 staff to 10 months. A total of 264 personnel are needed to adequately staff the new facility.

"The U.S. government cannot spend over $25 million of the taxpayer's money for a new facility and then leave it half empty," Zah said.

The proposed cuts are the of executive orders fron Clinton Administration to r the costs of the fe government by elimin 252,000 jobs in three year to cut administrative costs federal agencies.

In addition to the fact health care on Indian reserv: has always been under-fu Zah said health care is a responsibility of the government.

B4 Wednesday, February 2, 1994

FOUR CORNERS — The Daily Times Farmington, New Mexico

Hospital without a staff?

MALCOLM BRENNER
STAFF WRITER

SHIPROCK — The Northern Navajo Medical Center, approaching completion on the hill north of town, is the state-of-the-art in health care technology.

With the structure 70 percent complete, Gary Brainard, with the Tucson design firm Anderson DeBartolo Pan, has been giving tours for the hospital's steering committee and guests like Navajo Vice President Marshall Plummer.

In the dark interior, Brainard pointed with pride to rooms still nothing more than spaces divided by steel studs.

"Nurses in this area will have control over the airflow," he said.

"If the patients have infectious diseases, the air will flow in, keeping their germs in. If they suffer from immune system diseases like AIDS, the air can be made to flow out, keeping germs out."

There will be four outpatient clinics, four surgical suites, four labor-and-delivery rooms, a 24-chair dental facility and dozens of private examination

... nice new hospital, ... we will ... improved

Notah

said.

The complex electro-mechanical controls in the new facility will require retraining for the operators and maintenance people.

Esthetics have not been forgotten.

Imported limestone was used for the walls.

The building is culturally appropriate, mimicking the lines and forms of Shiprock, and oriented towards the east.

Even a hogan has been included on the grounds for traditional ceremonies.

With its own power and heating systems, the 225,000 square-foot building — double the size of the old hospital — will be what engineers call a "stand alone" facility.

Hospital administrators wor-

Peterson Zah can convince Bill Clinton to cancel planned cutbacks in IHS staffing, the $32.5 million hospital will be "standing alone" when it opens in September — severely understaffed.

Dee Hutchison, the hospital's chief executive officer, said the NNMC, if fully staffed, would employ over 1,000 people — double the current employment.

"We would have a nice new hospital, but with no new staffing we will not be able to provide an improved level of service," said IHS spokesperson Jenny Notah.

"The new facility will not be utilized to the maximum benefit if we have insufficient staff" Notah said.

Attempts are being made to

services.

Ron Wood, with the IHS Area Office in Window Rock, said that IHS headquarters and area-level offices will take "more than their share of cuts" in administration, travel and support positions, leaving service units unaffected.

But Hutchison said "cuts will be across the board, from clinical to administrative support."

Notah said staff might be asked to take a 2-day furlough without pay to make ends meet.

One solution is to contract out services lost in the cuts.

Notah — and some doctors — don't think that will reduce costs. Contracted services are two to three times more expensive than payrolled employees, Notah said.

If contracting is necessary, Hutchison said the Navajo tribe would be given the first option.

The paradoxical situation has administrators and staff worried.

No one seems to be sure what will happen next.

"It's ridiculous for us to be that short of staff, going into a new facility," said one staffer who asked not to be identified.

Cutbacks threaten hospital staffing

MALCOLM BRENNER
STAFF WRITER

SHIPROCK — Suppose the U.S. government gave the Navajo Tribe a brand-new hospital, and no staff to work in it?

That is the situation confronting Shiprock's health-care community as the Northern Navajo Medical Center nears completion.

"The hospital is like a dream becoming reality, yet other mandates are coming from President Clinton and Congress," said Dee Hutchison, the hospital's chief executive officer.

In April, Clinton ordered cuts of 100,000 jobs from the federal work force. Some of them are coming out of the Indian Health Service.

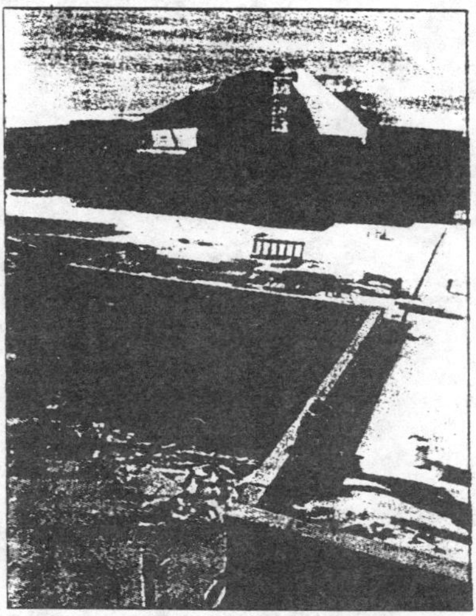

Malcolm Brenner/The Daily Times
The Northern Navajo Medical Center, nearing completion, has been designed to echo the shapes and forms of Shiprock.

"Initially, the IHS requested positions for the new hospital in the fiscal year 1995 budget," said Jenny Notah, spokesperson for the Navajo area IHS.

In addition to the 520 full-time and 40 part-time staff employed at the old hospital, 264 new full-time jobs were planned for the new facility, Hutchison said.

Then, just before Christmas, hospital administrators learned that the cutbacks would mean no new staff for the new hospital.

"There is no budget for new staffing," Notah said. "We were told to maintain employment at the current level. For FY 1995 there would be no increases for positions for facilities scheduled to open in 1995, including Shiprock."

Currently there are between 3,200 and 3,300 full-time equivalent (FTE) positions in the Navajo area IHS, Notah said. Current plans call for cutting back to 3,041 by Oct. 1994 and 2,977 by Oct. 1995.

As a consequence, the new Shiprock hospital, which is scheduled to become operational in September, may be required to lay off as many as 105 positions from current staffing.

An empty wonder of technology
Page B4

Hutchison said that recent changes in IHS staffing methodology, based on workload, now call for 515 FTE positions at the new hospital, rather than the 264 originally planned for.

"Essentially, the service unit is trying to provide an increased level of service with the same number of staff," Notah said. "The new facility will not be utilized to maximum benefit with insufficient staff."

The result, Notah said, would be that some space would end up not being used.

Navajo President Peterson Zah is scheduled to meet this morning with Ira Magaziner, President Clinton's chief White House aide for health reform, in an attempt to resolve the staffing problem.

"The U.S. government cannot spend over $25 million of the taxpayer's

Thursday, August 26, 1993

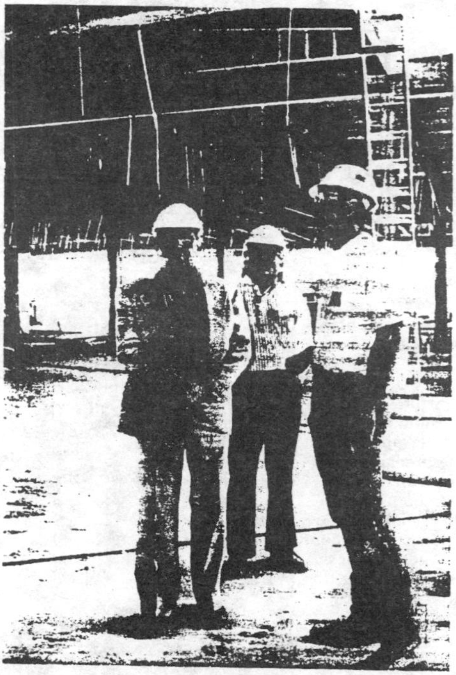

President Zah and staff assistant Charley John tour the construction site of the new Shiprock health care facility with project manager Centex Bateson. (Photo by Kenji Kawano)

New Shiprock health facility on schedule

SHIPROCK - Construction of the new Shiprock Comprehensive Health Care Facility is on schedule for completion in 1994 and the workforce has averaged 77 to 80 percent Navajo.

Last Thursday, Navajo Nation President Peterson Zah toured the construction site of the $50 million facility. The project is now 50 percent complete.

Zah was pleased that the project has a good working relationship with the Office of Navajo Labor Relations, the tribal office which works to ensure that tribal labor laws are followed.

"In addition to meeting the great need for a new hospital for the area, the project is providing jobs for Navajo people," Zah said.

In phase one of the construction which is currently underway, Navajos make up 149 of the total workforce of 199. The 15 subcontractors for the project also provide training when they cannot find qualified Navajo workers.

Gloria Harrision, member of the Shiprock Hospital Steering Committee, said the new hospital will be three times larger than the old facility which was built 1959 and opened in 1960.

325-4545 The Daily Times Friday, November 13, 1992

Hospital builders moving earth

MALCOLM BRENNER
STAFF WRITER

SHIPROCK — Moving 36,000 cubic yards of earth as they prepare the site, the construction crew at the new PHS Shiprock Indian Hospital is racing against the changing seasons.

Should extreme cold set in before the vertical concrete slabs forming the walls are poured, the work could be delayed.

Chris Robinson, project manager for prime contractor Centex-Bateson of Dallas, is optimistic.

"We're on schedule. I don't foresee any problems or delays," he said.

From sunrise to sunset, huge machines called scrapers roll back and forth over the 20-acre site just east of the current hospital.

They scrape hundreds of cubic yards of dirt from one area and spread it over another, leveling the ground.

Then comes a water truck, wetting the dirt for better compaction.

It is followed by a steamroller-like machine called a sheeps foot compactor.

The process, Robinson said, involves turning the soil into a series of lifts, or layers, that will provide a firm base for the hospital's 216,000-square foot concrete slab foundation.

Another 28,000 cubic yards of fill will be brought in, raising the level of the site eight feet.

Backhoes are digging trenches for utility mains. Pouring the foundation slab is set to start in about 10 days.

The site is not hiring presently, but Robinson said that if the weather cooperates, more workers will be needed when the pouring begins.

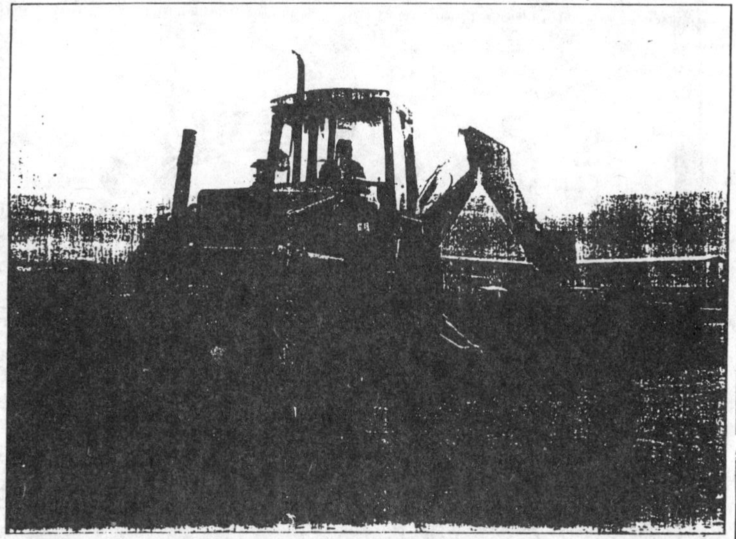

Malcolm Brenner staff photo

A backhoe operator works at the construction site of the new PHS Shiprock Indian Hospital. Construction crew members working with one eye on the weather.

NAVAJO NATION
DIVISION OF HEALTH

Department of Behavioral Health Services
Testimony
on

Navajo Nation Health Issues:
Alcohol/Substance Abuse/Mental Health

TESTIMONY OF NORMAN RATION, DIRECTOR

NAVAJO NATION DIVISION OF HEALTH

DEPARTMENT OF BEHAVIORAL HEALTH SERVICES

before

HONORABLE SENATOR PETE DOMINICI

HONORABLE SENATOR JOHN McCAIN

HONORABLE CONGRESSMAN JOHN KYLE

TOPIC:

NAVAJO NATION HEALTH ISSUES

ALCOHOL/SUBSTANCE ABUSE/MENTAL HEALTH

SHIPROCK, NEW MEXICO

APRIL 8, 1994

TESTIMONY ON NAVAJO NATION ALCOHOLISM PROBLEMS
Shiprock Field Hearing
Shiprock High School Gymnasium
APRIL 8, 1994

INTRODUCTION

Good afternoon, Honorable Senator McCain, Honorable Senator Domenici, Mr. President, Members of the Tribal Council and distinguished guests: Thank you for the invitation to offer testimony today at this important hearing.

My name is Norman Ration and I am the Acting Director of the Navajo Nation Department of Behavioral Health Services, Division of Health. I am honored and pleased to offer testimony on behalf of approximately 55,000 alcohol and drug afflicted Navajo population who are suffering and struggling with their lives to combat these diseases (DBHS Annual Report, 1992). I have been delegated the responsibility to present evidence of a serious health crisis affecting our Navajo people, both male and female, youth, adults and elders. This is a grave issue because our people are seriously ill, physically, mentally and spiritually and are dying in very disproportionate numbers due to alcoholism and lack of appropriate resources to overcome this problem. As a Navajo and having been employed with the human services programs for the past years, I have witnessed and experienced the harassment, intimidation, discrimination and indifference toward our Navajo people for being alcoholics and/or drug addicts. Now is the time for awareness and compassion for the afflicted who can become productive citizens once again.

The Navajo DBHS provides and coordinates alcohol treatment programs through five agencies and several field offices in a geographic area 27,000 square miles in size. Individual and group outpatient treatment and counseling services are provided to clients, youth, and adults whose lives are affected by alcohol and substance abuse and associated problems. These five (5) agency centers are located in Tuba City, Chinle, Fort Defiance, Crownpoint, and Shiprock and five-sub-offices which are located in Newlands, Page, Kayenta, Dilcon, and Window Rock. A unique feature of the treatment provided is the use of methods blending traditional and western health models. Services using traditional ways of healing to DBHS active clients has proven to be a positive attribute of the program. (See Exhibit "A1" and "A2"-DBHS Abstracts.)

However, none of these programs effectively deal with the high-risk environment to which the abuser returns. Pre- and post-treatment procedures developed and linked to a treatment program for each client do not work due to lack of follow-up. Further, services are hindered by weak networking, lack of effective aftercare mechanisms, huge distances and multiple jurisdictions. Denial on the part of the abusers, rural isolation of clients, and foremost, lack of treatment facilities are major barriers to effective treatment programs. In addition, there are insufficient numbers of detoxification beds or facilities available on the reservation. The Indian Health Service (IHS) hospital facilities have limited or no provision for medical detoxification on the reservation.

I. STATISTICAL INFORMATION

In general, the health status of the Navajo population is poorer than that of the United States population. The poor health status of the Navajo population is to a great extent related to the low standard of living and/or environmental factors. According to the 1990 census, the average annual per capita income of all persons on the Navajo Nation is far below that of the U.S. average. Less than 50% of the homes have piped water and waste facilities and only about one in seven homes have a telephone (1990 Census). The health problems of the Navajo people range from acute, infective and parasitic diseases to chronic neoplasms and congenital anomalies (IHS report, 1992).

The infective/parasitic diseases stem to a large degree from unsanitary water and sub-standard living conditions. Obesity is a serious nutritional problem and is linked to the diet of the Navajos which is high in starch and fat. Although no casual link has been established between energy-related environmental factors and chronic problems such as cancer and respiratory conditions, there is a higher prevalence of these diseases in areas of significant energy development. Various studies indicate that <u>alcohol is one of the major contributing factors to morbidity and mortality in the disease categories listed below as leading causes.</u>

1. Accidents
2. Disease of the Heart
3. Pneumonia and Influenza
4. Homicide
5. Diabetes Mellitus
6. Cerebral Vascular Diseases
7. Suicide
8. Chronic Liver Disease and Cirrhosis
9. Congenital Anomalies

SPECIAL TARGET POPULATIONS

Several sources indicate that Navajo Women are underserved. Their specific health needs, especially alcohol related health problems have not been addressed adequately. Teen health pregnancies are on the rise. Prenatal and postpartum services are limited. As a result many Navajo women are not receiving these services. IHS, the other major service provider on the Navajo Nation, provides limited services focused on women's needs and has observed that the Navajo woman is becoming a high-risk group for alcohol-related birth defects or Fetal Alcohol Syndrome (FAS). Additionally, a survey of women seen in a five-state IHS psychiatric service center showed that 80% experienced some sort of sexual assault. Third (3rd) among specific leading causes of Navajo female deaths was motor vehicle accidents, many attributed to alcohol.

Based on various sources, Navajo youth aged 12-18 and young adults aged 19-35 (especially male) are in the high risk group. In any given community on the reservation and bordertown communities, the use of drugs, alcohol and other substance abuse is evident. An IHS 1991 report indicated 25.2% or more than 1/4 (one fourth) of 22,080 total population of this high risk group have experienced the use of alcohol, marijuana and inhalants. The report further indicates that the use of alcohol and drugs by 8th grade Navajo and other Indian students off the reservation is 35.0%. Therefore, the importance of providing comprehensive treatment to this age group through direct service programs is essential. Very little or limited service on alcohol and drug abuse is being provided to these youth/adolescents in school and dormitory settings on the reservation and surrounding communities.

II. FACILITIES

Currently, off-reservation residential treatment facilities have been identified & are utilized - however, these facilities are very expensive and insufficient as to cultural sensitivity and relevancy, besides being distant from the reservation. It is our goal to provide treatment for the Navajo closer to home where they can maintain domestic ties. We feel that residential treatment centers within the boundaries of the Navajo Nation will better serve the needs of our people as compared to urban settings which are often the source of substance abuse.

Border towns are grossly affected by the lack of reservation facilities. A prime example of border town affliction is Gallup, NM. A review of high risk client data indicates Navajo communities around Gallup, New Mexico are severely impacted by chronic alcoholism. (See Exhibit "B"-Na'Nizhoozhi Center (NCI), Target Population) These are communities where there are no existing services at present. Analysis of high risk data indicates that currently 594 individual clients also represent 49.2% of all Protective Custody admits.

This is only one indication of an immediate need for intense and structured services for chronic Navajo alcoholics; short-term and long-term rehabilitation, halfway houses and custodial care. Navajo communities need immediate implementation of treatment of high risk alcoholism and outpatient services for intervention. The tribal government has now recognized that the current client-centered treatment programs operated predominately off-reservation or scattered across a large geographic area have had only limited success. Most Navajo clients who go away to treatment, return to an unchanged environment and resume former patterns of behavior.

Specific studies that have been conducted on the Navajo Nation throughout the years have come to the general conclusion that much of the Euro-American modalities for treating substance abuse are problem-oriented, client-centered approaches which have had little success in treating Native Americans. Both scholars and tribal representatives point out that holistic approaches are needed that target families and individuals at all age levels. This community-based approach would address the unique social and cultural circumstances in the Navajo reservation communities.

Recognizing that environmental characteristics impact patterns of abuse in Navajo communities, the tribal government intends to heighten community awareness of the problem and create the necessary community mobilization together with enhanced program and service delivery infrastructure to address the problem. The tribal government envisions a network of community directed treatment and prevention programs utilizing a holistic and multidisciplinary model, which will support healing and health in Navajo communities.

As an example, the Crownpoint Department of Behavioral Health Services has been an effective outpatient component in our campaign against substance abuse integrating a holistic family support system to strengthen client rehabilitation. This effectiveness is being compromised by the lack of adequate residential facilities, a situation which we have and are still trying to remedy with funding requests from foundations and a small grants from IHS for piece-meal renovation. This effort is requiring immediate attention, because by our creating culturally sensitive treatment facilities, we would realize a significant reduction in substance abuse, and encourage cost savings not only in dollars, but also in human suffering.

In the interests of promoting the health and welfare of the Navajo people, we strongly support the proposed reservation based drug and alcohol treatment facilities. We want to sustain and prolong the life of our people who can benefit from this development. The proposed residential treatment facilities on the Navajo Reservation will have several specialized units including a unit for mental health patients which is now becoming a precedent and recognized as part of overall well being.

The dire need for treatment facilities has been thoroughly and emphatically discussed by DBHS, NNAIHS and other local and regional entities who have experienced the Navajo alcoholism problem first hand. The consensus of all concerned cites these areas of recommendations and are confirmed in a memo dated March 31, 1994 (See Exhibit "C".)

1. There is a need for a medical and/or social setting detoxification center on the Navajo Reservation, as hospital beds are usually not available for such services unless the patient's condition is serious and requires

intensive medical detox services. In addition to this center is the need to have a Pre-treatment Component, to assist a patient entering a residential or outpatient program.

Along with the aforementioned, is the need for a short-term residential treatment program and/or intensive outpatient program, coupled with a strong community-based aftercare program for the importance of quality Continuum of Care for the patients and family who are provided services.

2. There presently exists, a gap in linkage of the Continuum of Care of aftercare services for the youth and also in the continuum of care of detoxification, residential, intensive outpatient, and aftercare services for the adults and family. Consistency in the service delivery is difficult to attain and maintain when there's fragmentation of service due to lack of facilities and resources.

3. We need available Halfway houses and Three Quarter houses for those homeless and in need of shelter. These living quarters would assist those in need of these services to make the necessary life adjustments in his/her life, to become productive citizens of our Nation again.

4. Larger facilities of emergency shelters for our abused children and families is a high priority on the Navajo Reservation. At the present time, such shelters house only a few mothers and children, while our child abuse, spouse abuse and violence associated with alcohol and/or substance abuse and dependencies are on a continual rise.

We collectively accede that these facilities are all priority needs for our Nation and request that it be treated as such in determining funding allocations. Delays or reductions in allocating these funds will further jeopardize lives. The Crownpoint project has proven on record its strives to rehabilitate but we need to expand on these services. Your cooperation in facilitating the identification and appropriation of treatment facilities would be appreciated.

III. PREVENTION AND EDUCATION

A preventive aspect also comes into play in the total continuum of client care. It is easier, as well as more cost-effective, to prevent alcoholism than it is to treat it. Early identification of alcohol abusers also leads to more cost-effective treatment, and so educational sessions directed at the community are conducted as part of DBHS operations although not at the comprehensive level we wish to. Prevention treatment efforts in the Navajo Nation cannot be successful when the environment is overwhelmed by the assessibility and glamorization of alcohol.

Prevention and education efforts are targeted mainly at children and adolescents through programs instituted in the schools. There are several school districts in the Navajo Nation which have some sort of alcohol education/prevention programs in place. In addition, there are several Bureau of Indian Affairs and mission schools. All of these schools have varied level of substance abuse prevention and education programs in place. However, they did not adequately address the needs of the adolescents. There must be more programs in place which will prevent future spread of abuse. A recent impromptu survey of Navajo 7th and 8th graders found that 17% of the adolescents came from households where there was a drinking problem and another 58% had one or more parents who were alcoholics.

Prevention of alcohol/drug abuse is the key component in the entire alcohol service program. The Department of Behavioral Health Services is struggling to develop a comprehensive preventive program to meet the needs of the Navajo people which will effectively deal with the high-risk environment to which the abuser must return. Presently, the programs provide piecemeal services needed to strengthen its weak networking, referral and aftercare mechanisms.

More effective medical, mental health, and legal intervention services are needed from community providers to ensure chronic alcoholics are further removed from their drinking cycles.

Thus, we adamantly confirm that:

> More dollars need to be granted for the prevention of alcohol and substance abuse in school settings and community based programs (with prevention efforts culturally specific and target population oriented); and that these dollars also be used to develop quality recreational centers for Alcohol and Substance Abuse Prevention (ASAP) activities throughout the Navajo reservation for the youths and families, e.g. properly maintained community indoor/outdoor basketball/tennis courts, softball/baseball fields, fitness centers, parks, etc.
>
> Note: Attachments Exhibit "D" - Memo dated 11-17-92, Subject: National Center for Substance Abuse Treatment, Washinton, D.C. visit and Exhibit "E" - Justification for FY1995 (Facility) Funding are attached to attest the submittals of these documents to various sources for funding with no positive response as yet.

IV. MENTAL HEALTH

Because of limited information specific to the Navajo Nation we rely on this study entitled "A Comprehensive Mental Health Care System for Native Americans in New Mexico" (See Exhibit "F"-) which is inclusive of the Navajo people

Findings from the Literature Review

American Indians represent 8.9% of the population of New Mexico. New Mexico has the fourth greatest number of Native Americans and the second largest percentage of any state. The Indian population of the State is the fastest growing ethnic group and by the time the ten-year planning/construction/implementation phases of this report are completed (2003), there will be 181,379 Indians in the State. This is a 35% increase. Therefore, estimates of need may also increase by a similar factor.

American Indian males suffer substantially higher rates of violent death than other groups in New Mexico. Such causes which are usually classified as parapsychiatric in nature include: motor vehicle crashes, other injuries, suicide, homicide, and other substance and alcohol-related problems such as cirrhosis of the liver, alcohol dependence syndrome, and alcoholic pychosis.

Fetal Alcohol Syndrome has become a problem among New Mexico Indians in the past 15 years, and it is, on average, twice as high among New Mexico Indians as among other people in the U.S.

The literature review yielded many studies relevent to American Indian mental health in the areas of: epidemiology (prevalence patterns, and overall causes of problems), individual mental health disturbances treated in clinics, and issues and models of service delivery.

Problem drinking indicators, depression, anxiety, marital problems, and situational disturbances are also the most commonly treated problems in both health and mental health clinics and hospitals serving American Indians in New Mexico. In one recent study alcohol problems accounted for 75% of inpatient mental health episodes at New Mexico IHS and contract hospitals and 52% of the Indian Health Service (IHS) outpatient episodes. Overall, 21% of New Mexico Indians of all ages will utilize an IHS facility for a mental health/substance abuse problem over a ten-year period. This, therefore, is a measure of treated prevalence.

Highlighted in the literature review of the report are a number of "ideal" or "model" programs known to the project planning staff which includes a need for increased cultural sensitivity to be used in mental health care, a need for increasing Indian access to care, and a need for training more Indian mental health professionals.

Finally, stakeholder interviews and focus groups of tribal and communities leaders and consumers were used to further define local concerns, issues and ideas. Special tribal cultural traits and community desires were assessed for further definition of appropriate needs and services.

Guiding Principles

Local, community-based care and services are always emphasized. Cooperation among spiritual, medical, and psychosocial healers will occur, along with the integration of the strengths of the extended family and community.

Some Additional Recommendations Made in the Plan

Legislative recommendations are made in the plan. State legislation which would give partnership to tribal mental health and substance abuse programs is needed. Furthermore, tribal court orders regarding involuntary commitments for mental health treatment should be discussed and resolved by Tribal and state representatives. Changes in state statutes might be needed to support the concept of culturally appropriate care for Indian youth and adults. Furthermore, IHS inpatient care contracts should contain provisions for cultural sensitivity in the provision of care. Policies and legislative provisions are needed to provide public and private recognition and benefits for traditional Native American healing practices as defined to be appropriate by each tribe.

The dire need for mental health treatment programs and facilities has also been thoroughly and emphatically discussed by DBHS, NNAIHS and other local and regional entities who have experienced the Navajo mental health problems first hand. The consensus of all concerned cites these areas of recommendations: (See Exhibit "G")

A summary of the services provided and needed in the area on Mental Health on the Navajo reservation has never been a "wealthy" program, and so the thought of "tightening our belts" in the spirit of government "reinvention" (while appealing in the abstract), is actually an insult to the intelligence of anyone truly aware of the conditions faced by our mentally ill or alcoholic community members. Unfortunately, the people most in need of our services - those with severe mental illnesses, those in need of residential alcoholic rehabilitation, and children in need of long-term treatment and supervision-are already poorly served in most cases.

1. There is no day treatment of any kind for severely mentally ill Navajo adults anywhere on the reservation except for Kayenta agency, where the program received one-time once-a-year funding through IHS Contract Health "left over" dollars from the end of fiscal year 1993. This program has already demonstrated major savings in the form of prevention of re-hospitalization for the patients receiving these services.

2. There is no clear avenue for the funding of long-term placement of children who, because of risky behavior (chronic suicidality, perpetration of sexual offenses, running away, drug abuse, truancy, etc.) require a placement more intensive than a foster or group home for an extended period of time. This is particularly true for the increasing number of children affected by Fetal Alcohol Syndrome with its associated impulsive behavior, poor social adjustment, and risk of substance abuse. There are not enough foster homes. Those families willing to provide homes are not trained or supported adequately due to a shortage of resources, and there are no therapeutic foster homes at all.

3. There is also no available inpatient pyschiatric service for adults or children on the Navajo Reservation. People needing this care are transported far from their homes and families to expensive, for-profit facilities where often no staff member even speaks Navajo.

4. Finally, the problems of alcoholism - medical, vocational, social, community, and in multi-generational and cultural self-esteem - are not being addressed as high priority despite political claims to the contrary. There is not a single comprehensive adult alcohol rehabilitation facility with available medical services anywhere on this reservation, the largest in the United States. This is an embarrassment to the IHS, the federal government, and the tribe.

We would invite the senators and any government representatives to visit the trailers and ramshackle buildings in which we provide services before deciding we can absorb reductions using creative "reinvention".

V. FUNDING REQUEST FOR A COMPREHENSIVE PREVALENCE STUDY (See Exhibit "H"-Proposal: Prevalence of Alcohol Abuse Among the Navajo submitted by Phillip A. May, Ph.D.)

The prevalence study of substance abuse among adults, particularly alcohol use and abuse, has not been well studied among many American Indian tribes or Alaska Natives. Nevertheless, with the exception of the two studies on the Navajo, there are few prevalence data available for Navajo which could be used to plan specific and targeted prevention or intervention programs for the Navajo Nation. As of 1989, only six published articles had reached print in major academic journals or books (see May, 1989a). Other studies have been done on alcohol use among Indian adults in other sites, but the data are not readily available or easily accessible.

Further, since tribes differ considerably from one another on a variety of behaviors, a study done on one reservation might not be too useful to another reservation or, even less useful to another tribe. Of the six published studies which involve Indian adults, two were done on the Standing Rock Sioux, two on the Navajo (main reservation), one on the Southern Ute and one on the Brokenhead Ojibway (in Canada). Most of these studies have used different criteria, the same methods differ, the results were reported in different ways and the time periods are very different (ranging from 1960 to 1984).

There have been a number of studies done on Navajo school children. These studies, and their results, are available in a variety of publications (see May, 1989a and 1982 for references). Researchers such as Oetting and Beauvais (1985), Winfree and Griffiths (1983) and a number of tribes and agencies have done a considerable amount of surveying in this category. These surveys have been put to use in creating school-based prevention programs in a variety of ways and in a variety of sites. Therefore, the prevalence of substance use and abuse among Indian school children is hardly an unstudied area, at least as far as surveys are concerned. <u>It is the adult and non-school youth (dropout) prevalence and patterns about which we know the least, or have the least data.</u>

The two published studies done among the Navajo were done by Levy and Kunitz (1974) and May and Smith (1988). In their book, <u>Indian Drinking</u>, Levy and Kunitz reported on studies done in 1969 among Navajos in four settings (two reservation areas, Flagstaff and hospital sample). They found that 30% of Navajos who were 18 years old or older drink at least once a year. Males were considerably more likely to drink than were Navajo females (52% versus. 13%). May and Smith did a stratified sample at the Winslow IHS Clinic in 1984 and found higher prevalence than the earlier Levy and Kunitz study; 52% of the Navajo sixteen years or older drank at least once a year (males = 64%, females = 40%). Therefore, the use of alcohol may be on the increase among the Navajo, particularly among females. Neither of these prevalence figures, however, are as high as the prevalence for the general U.S. but both studies, however, found that there were a substantial number of very heavy alcohol users within the Navajo drinking population, and that this proportion of problem drinkers was two to three times as great as among the general U.S. studies. None of the heaviest drinking alcohol abusers and alcoholics could be accessed in school studies.

Most studies which have tried to address the epidemiological features of Indian and Navajo drinking have done so by using indirect measures. Measures of mortality, morbidity, arrest and protective custody are commonly used to measure the magnitude and nature of the problem. But these are not the best measures of true prevalence and incidence. They are merely outcome measures, generated to a substantial degree by the problem drinking segment of the population; and they tell us little about the nature of the drinking patterns of the overall Navajo population. Further, with the exception of the mortality measures, these data are in most cases duplicative counts. That is, one person can generate many episodes of illness, arrest and protective custody, and the data make it appear as if a large number of individuals have the same problem when in fact it may be a real minority of the Navajo population at any one time. Many beliefs supporting the "Drunken Indian Stereotype" and inadequate prevention programs are often perpetuated because of poor prevalence data, incomplete knowledge and inaccurate information (see May, 1989a). A prevalence study will define the accuracy of a variety of beliefs.

Therefore, a prevalence of drinking survey among a particular tribe as the Navajo is a rare and promising study. Such a survey among the adult population will allow a tribe:

1. to identify the true extent of the problem,
2. locate the traits and types of individuals who are at greatest risk for alcohol abuse, and
3. to plan very specific and targeted treatment and prevention programs which are most appropriate for their people.

Such a study for and of the Navajo should be of tremendous utility for the future.

EXHIBIT "A1"

ABSTRACT

1994 CONTINUATION APPLICATION
(P.L. 94-437)

I. PROJECT DESCRIPTION

This grant continuation application requests funding from the Navajo Area Indian Health Service under the mandates of P.L. 93-638, the Indian Self-Determination Act to receive funds authorized by P.L. 94-437 (Health Improvement Act). The proposal is in response to formal notification of the availability of the Fiscal Year 1994 funding for Substance Abuse and Alcoholism services on the Navajo Nation through the Indian Health Service. The period for this funding reapplication is requested for a twelve (12) month period from January 01, 1994 through December 31, 1994.

The budget and justification are detailed under the Budget Section. The budget for the Behavioral Health Services totals $ 5,857,711. The budget will employ 150 people to carry out the Scope of Work.

The 1994 continuation application for P.L. 94-437 funds focuses on development of local communities to mobilize their efforts in combatting alcohol and substance abuse. In 1993 the Navajo Nation Department of Behavioral Health Services focused on seven (7) goals:

1) **Continuum of Care:** To provide a holistic comprehensive and effective alcohol and substance abuse treatment services to the adults and their families of the Navajo Nation.

2) **Traditional Healing:** To provide Traditional Treatment Services to adults and their families to restore harmony and balance through a holistic concept as an integral healing process.

3) **Corrections Project:** To facilitate spiritual and cultural Counseling and Support Services to Navajo and Native American Inmates in correctional facilities in Arizona, New Mexico, Utah and the Navajo Nation.

4) **Alcohol Women's Initiatives:** To support and promote prevention activities focusing on women.

5) **Quality Assurance:** To institute a quality assurance plan that insures quality care and an optimal level of services are rendered.

6) **Staff Development:** To encourage and provide staff development opportunities through cost effective, comprehensive training, education and certification programs to build and improve individual professionalism.

7) **Administration/Database:** To analyze, develop and implement a coordination of funds, resources and program development.

Continuum of Care

Outpatient counseling service activities to be rendered on a daily basis shall encompass family treatment services imperative to the success of the recovering client. The individual counseling activities will also be emphasized. Other important components include:

a. Screening and Evaluation
b. Referral process
c. Case Management
d. Assistance Services
e. Quality Assurance

Residential Treatment services will be continued and provided for adolescents and adults. The DBHS field offices will continue to assist adults and adolescent clients in residential treatment placements through border town settings and private facilities.

Outreach services shall serve as a vital part in which potential clients and/or their families are able to reach out for help. Outreach services shall enlist the originating process of incoming referrals providing intensive detailed assessments and progress information relative to service delivery, availability of treatment services and client confidentiality.

Aftercare services will be an important component within the continuum of care. Aftercare services for individuals, group and families will be provided by DBHS staff, including aftercare group and family sessions. Appropriate prevention education will be part of the aftercare services.

The Fetal Alcohol Syndrome (FAS) Prevention program is a comprehensive effort intended to reduce alcohol related birth defects. The Department of Behavioral Health Services will utilize a strong public media campaign in continuing its education and community awareness of FAS. FAS services will be provided by skilled and certified prevention specialist in the field offices.

The educational process will not be limited to FAS/FAE identification and treatment of at risk women on the Navajo Nation, but will include provision of technical assistance to other Navajo Nation service organizations.

Traditional Healing

This component shall be established to provide traditional and culturally integrated treatment (healing) services. Services shall include traditional healing ceremonies, traditional counseling methods and culturally relevant activities.

This component is unique in which western treatment methods and traditional methods will be integrated as part of the recovery process for individual clients. The emphasis shall be Navajo culture and traditions and some traditional healing will be provided by trained individuals with vast knowledge of Navajo traditions and culture. Healing ceremonies shall be provided by respected traditional medicineman from respective communities.

Corrections Project

The purpose is to provide a liaison between the Native American inmates, their families communities and Tribal Government. The project has a primary responsibility of assurin Navajo inmates and their families are afforded the opportunity to receive counselin sessions (individual, group and family) and participate in traditional ceremonies.

The project will research issues, identify and address the spiritual, cultural and lega needs of Navajo inmates in correctional institutions/facilities.

Alcohol Women's Initiative

The Department will provide support for prevention activities focusing on women, suc as:

a. Travel to relevant conferences/seminars;

b. Additional training to counselors and other staff on women's specifi treatment and prevention needs.

c. Support local training/conferences; and

d. Assist group development on women's substance abuse prevention an wellness.

Quality Assurance

The Department with the Division shall institute a quality assurance plan to ensure tha quality services are provided for all clients. The Department shall update and revise th existing quality assurance plan and standards.

Further, the Department shall establish a Quality Assurance Team to implement, monito and assess the quality assurance plan and standards. The Quality Assurance Team shal provide qualitative reviews, quantitative reviews and clinical case studies to ensure tha quality services are rendered.

Staff Development

The Department will continue to emphasize staff development activities in building a higl caliber staff of professionals. Staff development will be encouraged and facilitate through the following:

a. To provide a continuum of training for DBHS employees in which trainin will be based upon needs identified in the career plan/assessment. Caree ladders and/or degree programs will be developed for each staff member.

b. To certify 100% of direct services providers and maintain thei certification.

c. To establish and implement an appropriate salary scale for DBHS staff tha commensurate with qualifications and is competitive.

In addition to theoretical instructions, practical opportunities shall be made available. Internships at various residential programs will be developed and incorporated into staff development plan.

A major objective of the Department will be to institute a Certification Board that will be based on the Navajo Nation, and which will certify direct services providers.

Administration/Data Base

The administrative objectives of DBHS are:

a. To secure funds and distribute according to demographics.
b. To establish a network of policy making and coordination.
c. To identify and explore funding sources for the development of at least one treatment facility on the Navajo Nation.

The data base system will continue to be developed and expanded into a comprehensive and centralized information system. Through an integrated, centralized data base, there will be a uniformed reporting system.

Some benefits of an integrated, centralized database are:

a. A unique client tracking system
b. Recorded and documented profile on chapters and other essential information.
c. Access to geographical/demographic information.

The reporting system will be used to determine, conduct and compile a variety of data analysis and research studies.

EXHIBIT "A2"

ABSTRACT

1994 IHS CONTINUATION APPLICATION
P.L. 99-570 (OMNIBUS DRUG ACT)

I. PROJECT DESCRIPTION

This continuation application requests funding from the Navajo Area Indian Health Service under the mandates of P.L. 93-638, the Indian Self-Determination Act to receive funds authorized by P.L. 99-570 (Omnibus Drug Act). The proposal is in response to formal notification of the availability of the fiscal Year 1994 funding for Substance Abuse and Alcoholism services on the Navajo Nation through the Indian Health Service. The period for this funding reapplication is requested for a twelve (12) month period from January 01, 1994 through December 31, 1994.

The budget and justification are detailed under the Budget Section. The budget for the Omnibus Program totals $3,192,826.00. The budget will employ 27 people to carry out the scope of work.

The 1994 continuation application for P.L. 99-570 focuses on development of local communities to mobilize their efforts in combating alcoholism and substance abuse. As with the FY'93 Scope of Work, the Navajo Nation Department of Behavioral Health Services will focus on the following four (4) goals which have been expanded to illuminate on the seriousness of this disease while relating to the Navajo people the successes which have been realized in diminishing this problem.

These funds are primarily directed towards the adolescent:

GOAL 1. Continuum of Care
GOAL 2. Traditional Healing
GOAL 3. Community Awareness/Mobilization
GOAL 4. Sub-Contracts

The FY'94 Scope of Work was reviewed and revised by the DBHS administration, agencies, and suboffices' staff members. The Scope of Work, Goals and Objectives and the complementing activities/tasks basically will not change; however, some of the objectives and activities have been combined, refined and/or eliminated to reduce redundancy. Objective statements and activities narratives were reworded for clarity and to improve readability.

GOAL 1: CONTINUUM OF CARE
TO PROVIDE COMPREHENSIVE AND WHOLISTIC TREATMENT FOR CHILDREN, YOUTHS, AND THEIR FAMILIES THROUGH THE CONTINUUM OF CARE, UTILIZING A SERVICE MATRIX OF 2880 UNITS PER DIRECT SERVICE STAFF.

As summarized below, the concept of Continuum of Care will be rendered through the programs of Short and Long Term Treatment; Crisis Intervention; Aftercare; Wellness; and Fetal Alcohol Syndrome (FAS) Prevention.

Comprehensive treatment services will be provided for all ages ranging from children, youths to adults and to families who are affected through the use of alcohol and substance abuse.

GOAL 2: TRADITIONAL HEALING

TRADITIONAL TREATMENT SERVICES SHALL BE PROVIDED TO RESTORE HARMONY AND BALANCE THROUGH A WHOLISTIC CONCEPT AS AN INTEGRAL PART OF THE HEALING PROCESS.

This component is established to provide traditional and culturally integrated treatment (healing) services. Services include ceremonies, traditional counseling methods and culturally relevant activities.

This component is unique in that Western treatment methods and traditional methods are integrated as part or the recovery process for individual clients. The emphasis is on Navajo culture and traditions. Traditional healing is provided by trained individuals with a vast knowledge of the culture. Healing ceremonies are provided by respected traditional medicinemen in respective communities.

GOAL 3: COMMUNITY AWARENESS/MOBILIZATION

TO PROMOTE, SUPPORT AND ASSIST 110 LOCAL COMMUNITIES IN THE DEVELOPMENT OF THEIR CAPABILITIES TO REDUCE THE HIGH INCIDENCE OF ALCOHOL AND SUBSTANCE ABUSE.

This program achieves its goal (s) through the involvement of the local communities in the Navajo Nation by orientating and training Local Community Support Groups (LCSG'S) on programmatic services/policies as well as training them to implement educational services within their respective communities or chapters. This training evolves from the needs assessments which were conducted at each agency.

GOAL 4: SUBCONTRACTS

TO SUBCONTRACT AND COORDINATE WITH TEN SUBCONTRACTS FOR COMMUNITY EDUCATION, AFTERCARE, REHABILITATION AND TREATMENT SERVICES.

The program's focus is to monitor and evaluate subcontractors for compliance with applicable Navajo Nation, and federal (IHS) regulations and laws. As a continual available resource, the program provides guidance and technical assistance to subcontractors on the provisions of the Subcontractors Reference Manual and on other administrative and financial component areas. A prime responsibility is the undertaking of Requests for Proposals (RFP's), and assisting in the negotiating and awarding of contracts.

EXHIBIT "B"

Na'Nizhoozhi Center (NCI)

Target Population

The Protective Custody (PC) program in the City of Gallup dates back to 1973, when public toxication was decriminalized in the State of New Mexico. The purpose of Protective Custc has been to remove public inebriates from the city streets and to safeguard them from overexp sure and other life-threatening conditions, by holding them overnight at the city jail and then l ting them back out within twelve hours.

It is the purpose of NCI's program, then, to impact this protective custody population by prov ing improved conditions for public inebriates in custody, lengthening their stay in an envirc ment conducive to positive change, and providing some linkage with communities and service:

Through the operation of the Na'nízhoozhí Center, it is proposed to provide basic, tempora and humane shelter and custodial care, emergency referral for medical treatment, preliminary a sessment and intervention, and preliminary referral to detoxification, treatment, and\or other se vices, for a one-to-three day period, for persons taken into Protective Custody.

This program focus is based on the uniquely voluminous numbers of public inebriates who a picked up in Gallup under present PC procedures (i.e., an average of 80 persons per day, or mc than 26,000 PC incidents per year). These numbers overwhelm the capacity of more clinic or extended programs, such as standard social detoxification and treatment programs. The cc per client-day of such services prevents any substantial impact on the present PC population the numbers served would be minuscule (less than ten percent) in relation to the need. The pr posed program, then, constitutes a "preliminary detoxification" service emphasizing safe a clean shelter, preliminary intervention, and referral to other treatment programs in the area.

The great majority of persons picked up for Protective Custody in Gallup are Native Americar most of whom are Navajo, and 97% of whom reside outside of Gallup. According to the City Gallup's "Protective Custody Summary by Location" covering 9,000 records selected from fc separate months in 1988, the majority of pick-up points centered around Gallup's bars and pac age liquor outlets, with the balance of cases spread out over 700 locations around the city. T annual report for NCI's first year of operation (a copy of which is included in the attachmen confirms these numbers.

Gallup is a community of approximately 20,000 people, and the only incorporated municipali within McKinley County. The community is situated on Interstate 40, 140 miles west of Alb querque. The close proximity of Gallup to the Navajo Reservation and Zuni Pueblo has ma the city a major trade center, serving a trade area of more the 15,000 square miles and a popul tion of some 120,000 people, most of them Native Americans. The Navajo Reservation is t largest in the United States, with a total of more than 200,000 members and a land area of 25,0 square miles - larger than the state of West Virginia. With a population of 65,800, McKinl County is made up predominantly of minorities (78.8%), with almost two-thirds of the county population being Native American, primarily Navajo. The median age of 22.2 years makes it t youngest of all counties in New Mexico. Fewer than 40% of the persons over the age of 25 ha completed high school; the per capita income is less than 40% of that of the United States; ai almost one-third of the families live below the poverty level. On the average, Native America in McKinley County have a 1980 per capita income of less than $2,500; almost half (48.5%) li below the poverty level. Estimates of the unemployment rate on the Navajo reservation rang (across the various communities and districts of the reservation) between 40% and 75%.

The influx of Native Americans into Gallup, combined with the prohibition of alcohol on t nearby reservations, has led to the nation's most serious and most visible abuse of alcohol. Ga lup has received a national reputation as "Drunk City", and the statistics of alcohol abuse in Ga lup and McKinley County are astounding.

Gallup has 61 liquor outlets, which exceeds New Mexico's quota system by more than 550%. Gallup's bars are usually filled with Native Americans, many of whom drink until unconscious. To protect these individuals from staggering onto the highway or railroad, or freezing to death, the City of Gallup has developed a system of "Protective Custody" (PC) - incarcerating the individual without criminal offense for up to 12 hours. However, Protective Custody only provides relatively safe haven for alcohol abusers for a short time, after which the abusers are released - whereupon the cycle repeats itself.

On an average weekday night, Gallup police will pick up and place in Protective Custody between 20 and 80 inebriated persons. On weekends, the number of PC's will swell to between 100 and 200.

As identified in the findings of the December 1988 Report for the City of Gallup by Harting Associates, Inc., "Plan to Provide Services to the Public Inebriate-Protective Custody", there are different categories of individuals who are described as representing the Protective Custody (PC) and Drinking in Public (DIP) populations include; the "street people" who are chronic alcoholics; binge drinkers who live on the reservation but who drink to excess on periodic visits to town, often on weekends; and those who periodically become intoxicated on the reservation as well as in town.

According to the Harting Report, some of the problems experienced by many of the individuals picked up for protective custody include: physical deterioration; long-term\uninterrupted intoxication; impaired thought processes; generalized anxiety; obsession with drinking; severe withdrawal symptoms; interpersonal hostility; physical\medical complications; alienation from family, friends, etc.; suicidal tendencies; psychiatric disturbance; bodily injury; and homelessness. It was the conclusion of the Harting Report that most of the individuals picked up for Protective Custody were in need of continued observation, assessment of their physical and psychological condition, and motivation to commit to some form of treatment.

In the eleven-year span 1977-1987, an average of over 29,000 Protective Custody cases per year were recorded - more, for example, than the entire state of Illinois. As reported by Harting Associates, the following summarizes what is known about these adult episodes of Protective custody:

1. The best estimate is that there are 5,000 to 8,000 individuals (with some estimates as high as 12,000, based on the City of Gallup's four-month study identifying more than 4,000 separate PC individuals) represented in the 29,000 episodes of PC.

2. Approximately 75 individuals (1 to 1 1/2 % of the total) represent over 13% (3;900) of the entries into PC.

3. The usual weekly breakdown for PC entries is:

   Weekdays (Monday - Thursday) 50
   Weekends (Friday - Saturday) 100
   Sundays...30
   Occasional weekends (ceremonials, holidays, paydays, etc.) 180

4. It is estimated that 97% of the PC's are non-residents of Gallup, with 66% being residents of New Mexico and 33% residents of Arizona. About 40% of the individuals were documented as coming from the following seven communities: Crownpoint (7.5%); Ganado (7.5%);

Churchrock (7.0%); Navajo (5.5%); Chinle (5.0%); Window Rock (4.0%); and Gallup (3.5%).

5. It is estimated that 81% of the PC individuals are males and 19% are females.

6. The majority of PC individuals are between 30 and 60 years of age.

7. The vast majority of PC individuals are Native Americans (85 - 90%).

8. On the average, the 29,000 episodes represent: 2,416 PC entries per month; 558 per week; and 79 per day.

Clearly, these statistics represent numbers of individuals which would totally overwhelm e\ the largest existing systems within the State of New Mexico for social-setting detoxificati short-term treatment and other programs along the continuum of care. Although the program the Na'nízhoozhí Center does not purport to meet every dimension of the overwhelming need does set forth a new approach at the "low end" of the intervention continuum (i.e., "prelimin: detoxification" services).

Further, although there does not exist an adequately comprehensive continuum of services wit the Gallup area, the preliminary detoxification center is seen as an absolutely necessary elem in breaking the cycles of widespread alcohol abuse and public inebriation described in this s tion.

At the recommendation of the New Mexico Behavioral Health Services Division, representati of the City of Gallup and of the Northwest New Mexico Council of Governments toured fi detoxification and treatment centers throughout New Mexico to gather information regarding operation of detox programs and the problems and issues encountered in the process. This t proved useful in assisting City and COG staff to design a "preliminary detoxification" progra It was found, in fact, that such a program did not exist in the state of New Mexico, and that unique need in the City of Gallup with regard to the numbers of public inebriates was unpar leled. In the case of each site visited, it was found that relatively expensive services (for exa ple, $60 to $300 per client per day) were being provided to a relatively low number of indivic als.

It was the conclusion of the City officials and staff that a system was needed in Gallup whi would represent the "low end" of the intervention continuum, offering services to a significan higher number of individuals at a much lower cost such that the present system of protective c tody could be eliminated. Such a foundational program, working with chronic alcoholics a binge drinkers to arrest the cycle of habitual and repeated public intoxication, could then be co plemented by a variety of treatment programs on the Navajo Reservation, in the City of Gall and at other accessible locations. It was this concept that lead to creation of the Na'nízhoo Center.

EXHIBIT "C"

DEPARTMENT OF HEALTH & HUMAN SERVICES Public Health Service

MAR 31

Memorandum

Date March 31, 1994

From Jayne T. Goodluck, Branch Chief
NAIHS Alcohol & Substance Abuse Program

Subject Information on Potential Senate Hearing per dated memo of 03/21/94

To John Hubbard Jr., Area Director
Navajo Area Indian Health Services

Per request per memo, I have the following information to report on the Navajo Area Indian Health Services, Alcohol & Substance Abuse Program:

ACCOMPLISHMENTS:

•1. Shiprock's Four Corners Regional Adolescent Treatment Center attained, and has maintained full JCAHO Accreditation since December 1992. The facility is one of 9 operating, U.S. IHS - National Congress mandated, P.L. 99-570 funded residential treatment centers for youths. (Attached is the listing for all RTC programs.) Shiprock FCRATC is a 90 day, 24 bed (16 males & 8 females) treatment center for Native Americans.

•At the present time, Shiprock FCARC's CDMIS data system is being seriously considered to be the model system, for other Regional Treatment Centers to duplicate and/or modify for implementation within their respective Area programs. Headquarters East & West Alcohol & Substance Abuse Program staff are consulting with Dallas Parga and other FCARC staff.

•2. Mid November 1993, the Navajo Nation, Navajo Division of Health, Department of Behavioral Health Services received a million dollar CSAT grant, to plan and develop a culturally competent outpatient/inpatient alcohol and substance abuse prevention and treatment program for citizens of the Navajo Nation. Their vision is to develop community mobilization initiatives by identifying and establishing 10 Community Alcohol/Substance Abuse Prevention Committees. The committees will comprise of community members who will then monitor Dine Center for Substance Abuse.

Within the past couple of months, the core of DSCAT Steering Committee formed and met twice. Ms. Bea Bowman, on IPA from Headquarters, will be assisting Navajo Nation DBHS and the DSCAT Steering Committee in the development of this project. The staff positions for this project are currently being advertised in the Navajo Times. The project is underway.

•3. Gallup Na'nizhoozhi Center, Inc. for the period of October 01, 1992 to January 31, 1994 provided services to a total of 9,792 individuals; total of 8,348 males and 1,444 females. (Copy of 02-14-94 report attached). Their current contract with the Navajo Tribe DBHS expires the end of June 1994.

•4. The Counselor Certification for Navajo Area is at 51%. Since certification of counselors has become a Congressional/legislative concern the past year, Navajo Area has made a committment to attain a higher percentage of certification among their staff, ensuring quality service delivery to patients and families of the Navajo Nation. (Copy of 1993 Area Program Counselor Certification report attached).

•5. Within the past year, 6-8 Primary Care Providers (Medical Staff) attended a brief chemical dependency orientation and workshop session, in Phoenix, Arizona. As a result, our clinics and hospital, will benefit in creating a more humane, supportive environment for our chemically dependent patients, and significant others. This awareness also supports the need for early ASAP intervention and prevention that could occur in the ER, TR and/or OPD of any clinic or hospital.

•6. With coordinated efforts and collaboration among many organizational people in Navajo Area and Regional areas, a Navajo Nation & Regional Areas Resource Directory was compiled and published the past year. This coming year will be the second publication of this directory. The directory includes a listing of chemical dependency programs, Social Services programs, Mental Health, Crisis and Emergency Shelters, and listing of Native American Consultants. The directory has a national mailing list of 200+ organizations.

•7. Navajo DBHS and NAIHS-ASAP have been working closely regarding the DCSAT project, counselor certification requirements, and scheduled site visits throughout Navajo Area. I believe this working relationship will continue in the future. Mr. Norman Ration, Ms. Loretta Canujo, and Central office staff have been helpful, the past year.

AREA OF CONCERNS:

•1. There is a need for a Medical and/or social setting detoxification center on the Navajo Reservation, as hospital beds are usually not available for such services unless the patient's condition is serious and requires intensive medical detox services. In addition to this center, is the need to have a Pre-treatment component, to assist a patient entering a residential or outpatient program.

•2. Along with the need of item# 1, is the need for a short-term residential treatment program and/or Intensive Oupatient program, and a strong community-based Aftercare program for the importance of Quality Continuum of Care for the patients and family, provided services to.

There presently, exists a gap in linkage of the continuum of care of Aftercare services for the Youth. In addition, therer exists a gap of linkage of the continuum of care of detoxification, residential, intensive outpatient, and aftercare services for the adults and family. Consistency in the service delivery is difficult to attain and maintain when there's fragmentation of services.

•3. A Halfway house; three quarter house availablity for those homeless and in need of shelter, is also needed. It would assist those in need of these services to make the necessary life adjustments in his/her life, to become productive citizens of our Nation again.

•4 Larger facilities of emergency shelters for our abused children and families is strongly needed on the Navajo Reservation. At the present time, such shelters house only a few mothers and children, yet our Child Abuse, Spouse abuse and violence associated with Alcohol and/or Substance Abuse and dependencies are skyrocketing high.

•5. More emphasis and dollars need to be generated for the Prevention of Alcohol and Substance Abuse in school settings and community based programs. The prevention efforts need to be culturally specific and target population oriented.

•6. More collaborative and cooperative efforts need to be facilitated by all agencies and systems within and outside of Navajo Area, on behalf of the well-being of our people. ("The right hand needs to know what the left hand is doing!") In doing so, there will be less duplication and territorialism.

•7. Prevention efforts -More emphasis needs to placed on the preciousness of our children and the invaluableness of our elders, to our native communities when it comes to any decision making on the livelihood of our people and Nation.

•8. *There is a need for quality Recreational Centers for ASAP prevention activities throughout Navajo Area, for the youths and families. i.e. Nicely maintained community indoor/outdoor basketball courts, softball/baseball fields, etc.............*

•9. *There's a need for a more positive, nurturing, and encouraging attitude on all Navajo Area service providers toward ASAP patients and family.*

•10. *Availability of Contract Health Care dollars for dual-diagnosed patients; alcohol and mental health, or other. And lastly, more funds for more staff. Most programs are understaffed and underpaid for the work they do.*

I'll be in my office Monday, should you have any questions or concerns. I can be reached at 505/ 368-2481/4971.

Respectfully Submitted.

cc: Dr. Douglas Peter, NAIHS CMO, PO
Norman Ration, NN DBHS
file

..DEPARTMENT OF HEALTH & HUMAN SERVICES

Public Health Service

Navajo Area
Indian Health Service
P.O. Box G
Window Rock, Arizona 86515-5004

March 21, 1994

Memorandum

To: *See Below

From: J. Hubbard, Area Director

Subject: Potential Senate "Hearing"

We have preliminary word that Senators McCain and Domenici may be in Shiprock on April 8, 1994 and want to hear from NAIHS Area Director as well as President Zah and the NDOH on several matters.

In the event the above takes place, it is likely my comments will have to be cleared by IHS-HQ and PHS and DHHS.

I won't know for certain what topics are to be covered until the last week in March. By copy of this memo, I'm asking each of the following to begin to prepare no more than a one-page outline and brief paragraphs of narrative for each topic on the outline as follows:

a) Hantavirus Update - Clinical:Dr. Allen Craig
b) Hantavirus Update - Environmental Health:Pat Bohan
c) Child Abuse Prevention Efforts: Abe Plummer/Dr. Diana Hu
d) AIDS: Richard Turner and Dr. Chris Percy
e) Substance Abuse: Jayne Goodluck and Dr. Peter
f) '95 Budget Comments: Ron Wood
g) Environmental Concerns (water/sanitaiton, open dumps)

I hope to narrow the focus somewhat by the end of March, but wanted some forewarning to go out so you can begin to prepare briefing materials (I'm not interested in "binders" on each subject) for my use.

PLEASE SUBMIT BY COB MARCH 30, 1994. THIS WILL ALLOW US TIME TO COMBINE REPORTS AND GET CLEARANCE.

Thanks to everyone in advance for your anticipated assistance.

John Hubbard Jr., Area Director
Navajo Area Indian Health Service

*ADDRESSEES
Dr. Allen Craig, Shiprock
Pat Bohan, OEHE
Abe Plummer, Mental Health/Soc. Services
Richard Turner, Area OEHE
Dr. Chris Percy, Shiprock
Jayne Goodluck, Shiprock
Ron Wood, Executive Officer
Dr. Peter, Chief Medical Office
Butch Dowell, OEHE
Dr. Diana Hu, Tuba City

Counselor Certification 1993

Area Programs

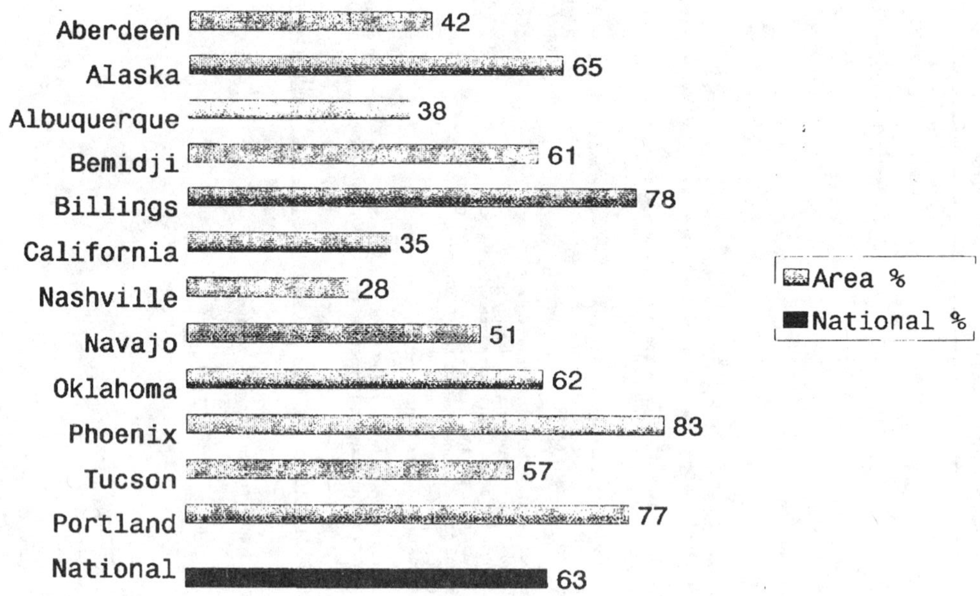

ASAPB-FB 1993

IHS YOUTH REGIONAL TREATMENT CENTERS

FNA/TCC Adolescent Treatment Program
Director: Ms. Florence Loucks
P.O. Box 74450
Fairbanks, AZ 99707
907/452-6925
FAX: 907/456-4849

Four Corners Adolescent Treatment Center
Director: Mr. Hoskie Benally
P.O. Box 567
Shiprock, NM 87420
505/368-4712
FAX: 505/368-5457

Inland Tribal Consortium Youth Treatment Center
Director: Ms. Claudia Flowers (Acting)
North 1617 Calispel
Spokane, WA 99205
509/327-9416
FAX: 509/327-9416

Jack Brown Youth Treatment Center
Director: Ms. Beverly Patchell
Cherokee Nation of Oklahoma
P.O. Box 948
Tahlequah, OK 74465
918/458-0496
FAX: 918/456-6485

Nanitch Sahallie Program
Director: Ms. Joanna Rogers
5119 River Road, NE
Keizer, OR 97303
503/390-5904
FAX: 503/390-6973

New Sunrise Regional Treatment Center
Director: Mr. Michael Smith
P.O. Box 219
San Fidel, NM 87049
505/552-6091
FAX: 505/552-6527

Phoenix/Tucson Youth Regional Treatment Center
Director: Annie Brayboy
P.O. Box 458
198 South Skill Center Road
Sacaton, Arizona 85247
602/379-3000 (Phoenix & Long Distance)
602/562-3801 (Sacaton Only)

Raven's Way
Director: Mr. Pat Hefley
222 Tongas Drive
Sitka, AK 99835
907/966-3061
FAX: 907/966-2259

Unity Regional Youth Treatment Center
Director: Dr. Mary Ann Farrell
P.O. Box C-201
Cherokee, NC 28719
704/497-3958
FAX: 704/497-6826

EXHIBIT "D"

THE
NAVAJO
NATION

P.O. DRAWER 308 • WINDOW ROCK, ARIZONA 86515 • (602) 871-4

PETERSON ZAH
PRESIDENT

MARSHALL PLUMI
VICE PRESIDENT

November 17, 1992

M E M O R A N D U M:

TO : Agency Directors/Department Directors

FROM : Alex Yazza, Acting Director
Department of Behavioral Health Services

SUBJECT: National Center for Substance Abuse Treatment, Washington DC Visit

A visitation was made by Lisa Sheckel from the National Center for Substance Abuse Treatment, Washington DC, on October 14 and 15, 1992. The purpose of the visit was to gain insight on present treatment facilities and the unmet needs of the Navajo people regarding Alcohol and Substance Abuse. The Department of Behavioral Health Services staff provided a tour which included the Shiprock Regional Treatment Center, Crownpoint Youth Crisis Intervention Center (CYCIC), and other proposed DBHS plans for treatment facilities.

According to Ms. Sheckel, there are funds available to renovate facilities and expand the needed services. As a result, a concept paper has been developed to give insight for a Comprehensive Campus Treatment Center on the Navajo reservation. Please, be cognizance that the concept paper is a rough draft. The Navajo Division of Health, Department of Behavioral Health Services will be responding to an RFP, coming down from the Washington office in March 1993.

Attached for your information is the concept proposal and the information provided by the Washington office regarding the proposed project. This information is being disseminated for all Departments and personnel who are expected to be involved in planning and implementation of proposed project.

cc: Doug Peters, Chief Medical Officer, IHS
Vivian Arviso, Staff Assistant, Office of the President
Charley John, Acting Director, NDOH

Ron Wood, Executive Officer, IHS
Harvey McKerry, Exec. Director, Division of Human Resources
Loretta Cunejo, ASO III, DBHS
George Etsitty, Planner, DBHS
Norman Ration, Assistant Director, DBHS
Roselyn Chapela, Planner, CHR
LaVerne Wyaco, Planner, NAAA
Madan Poudel, Planner, NDOH
James Sandoval, Agency Director, Crownpoint DBHS
Gene Johnson, Agency Director, Chinle DBHS
Rita Oquita, Acting Agency Director, Shiprock DBHS
Mattie Jensen, Fort Defiance DBHS
Agnes Dale, Tuba City DBHS
David Tsosie, Executive Director, Community Development

CONCEPT PAPER

NAVAJO DIVISION OF HEALTH'S PRIORITY PROJECT
Department of Behavioral Health Services

A. PRIORITY : **Navajo Nation Alcohol & Drug Abuse Treatment Center**

B. AGENCY : **Navajo Division of Health/Department of Behavioral Health Services**

C. AUTHORIZATION: IHS (Indian Health Services)
HUD (Housing, Urban & Development)
DHHS (Dept. of Health & Human Services)
CSAT (National Center for Substance Abuse Treatment)

D. APPROPRIATION: Federal appropriation's will be used for the development of Navajo Nation Alcohol and Drug Abuse Treatment Center.

E. ACTIVITY:
The treatment center will provide basic substance abuse counseling, Family Counseling, in and outpatient treatment, Health Education, Day Care services for children of dependent mothers, Family Intervention, Community Rehabilitation, Case Management, Outpatient/Aftercare Crisis Intervention, Community Education, Recreation/Physical, Mental Health Care,(FAS) Fetal Alcohol Syndrome Treatment, Cultural Healing and educational opportunities for clients coming out of continuum care program. Educational opportunities will be afforded through the Navajo Department of Employment & training Jobs Programs/JTPA, local high schools and Navajo Community College. Agreements will be established with various educational institutions and job training programs to entice clients to complete high school/GED, job training to become useful citizen in society.

F. REQUESTED AMOUNT: $30 million

CURRENT PROGRAMS:

Currently there are (11) eleven subcontractors who provid Services in Alcohol/Substance Abuse on and off th reservation. six (6) of the 11 subcontractors are locate on the reservation and (4) four facilities are locate outside the reservation. In addition there are (9) DBE service providers located in each of the agencies on th reservation who also provide services. However, th services provided fall short of needed services. Accordir to the 1988 Navajo Nation Fax, with the projected Annua growth rate of 2.48%, the total population of the Nava clients is 181,742. The total number of client being serve today Total 71,078. There are approximately 55,000 who a in need of immediate services. As the number of client increase, the demand for services is expected to increase

H. FEASIBILITY:

The priority for NDOH/DBHS is to develop adequate treatme facilities on the Navajo Nation. The Navajo Nation Department of Behavioral Health Services strongly emphasizes the need for comprehensive service delivery system that meets the need of the Navajo youth and adul members. Only through a local treatment center, which accessible and culturally relevant, will the Nation beg effectively dealing with the disastrous consequence of alcoholism and substance abuse. In addition, many Nava people have indicated they want facilities established or near their own communities. NDOH/DBHS has begun to ta the initiative to develop plans for long term treatmen facilities and develop a strategic plan for development the near future. The NDOH/DBHS plans to work with priva providers who have the expertise and skills to operate lc term treatment facilities. The provision of this relationship would offer the Navajo Nation licensure ar certification capabilities to provide high standards oi care and treatment for Navajo youth and adults. The NDOH/DBHS will in effect become the long term treatme provider and will expand into new job opportunities, educational training for counselors, therapists, administrators, and professional staff.

NEED STATEMENT:

Despite numerous efforts being made to address the probl related to alcohol and substance abuse the problems continues to effect the lives of Navajo youth and adul The Navajo Nation encompasses approximately 25,000 squ miles of trust land within the States of Arizona, New Mexico and Utah. According to the Navajo Nation Government, the population estimate is approximately 170,000 with a median age of 19.3 and the rate of growtł 2.5% per year.

The Navajo Criminal Justice Information System has prepared a five year summary report 1986-1990 which reflects that Crownpoint Agency is the leading agency in incidence/offenses related to alcohol. Alcohol related incidence/injuries reflect that high risk ages of offenders fall in the age group, 20-29 of male population and the second highest is the 30-39 age group.

The Navajo Area Indian Health Service profile indicates that Gallup, Tuba City, Crownpoint, Shiprock and Fort Defiance Agency continues to maintain the highest rate of alcohol-related deaths, years of productive life lost due to alcoholism, and hospital discharges related to alcoholism and drug.

The IHS profile also reflects that 60% of all motor vehicle accidents and fatalities are alcohol-related on the Navajo Nation. The highest death rate related to alcohol falls in the age category of 25-34. This represents 33% of all deaths.

OBJECTIVE:

The objective is to submit a proposal, to the National Office of Substance Abuse Center and Mental Health Administration, Washington, DC., for the amount of thirty million dollars ($30 million) for the construction and development cost of proposed Navajo Nation Alcohol and Drug Abuse Treatment Center. The Proposed Treatment Center will accommodate the needed treatment center for the Navajo youth and adults and further rectify the problems identified in the need statement. In addition an instrument will be developed to link the Treatment Center to various Educational Agencies to further provide an opportunity to place clients on a program which will enable clients to obtain education and job skills. This a vital instrument in placing clients back into the mainstream of society as useful citizen. As funding is identified and secured, funds will be earmarked and appropriated to NDOH for construction and development.

ADDITIONAL FUNDS FOR CONSTRUCTION/OPERATIONS:

A strong effort will be made to seek all available funding sources to make this project a reality. The Navajo Division of Health, Planning and Development office is actively seeking all available funding sources which include the Community Development Grant, Department of Housing and Urban Development (HUD), Department of Health and Human Services (DHHS), private foundations that provide funds for construction and development.

ABSTRACT

PROJECT NAME: The Navajo Nation Alcohol & Drug Abuse Treatment Center

APPLICANTS: Larry Curley, Executive Director
Navajo Nation Division of Health

Alex Yazza, Acting Director
Department of Behavioral Health Services

ADDRESS: P.O. Drawer 709
Window Rock, Arizona 86515

ACTIVITIES: The Navajo Nation Alcohol & Drug Abuse Treatment Center will provide services including central intake, approximately (5) residential service delivery units, community based continuum care, mental health care, job training and educational remediation.

CAPACITY: One Central Intake Facility and approximately (5) Residential Service Delivery Unit.

PURPOSE: To construct and develop infrastructure tc facilitate for the needs of service delivery as identified in the need statement.

FEATURES: The Treatment Center will provide basic substance abuse counseling, in and out patient treatment, Health Education, Day Care Service, Family Intervention, Community Rehabilitation, Case Management, Outpatient After Care, Crisis Intervention, Community Education, Mental Health Care, Recreation/Physical Activities and Cultural Healing.

TOTAL COST ESTIMATE: $30 Million

FUNDS REQUESTED: $30 Million

NAVAJO NATION ALCOHOL & DRUG ABUSE TREATMENT CENTER

CHINLE, ARIZONA

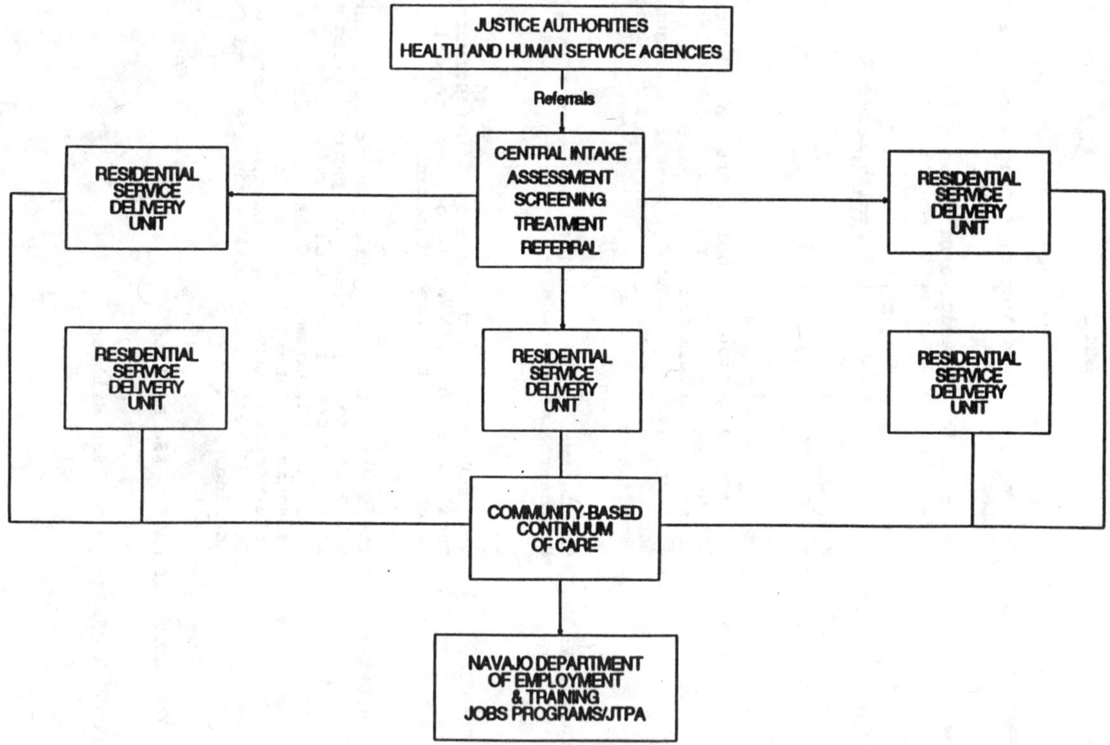

EXHIBIT "E"

JUSTIFICATION FOR FY 1995 FUNDING

Agencies	No. of Chapters	Approximate Population
Chinle	15	22,993
Shiprock	21	26,230
Crownpoint	31	27,458
Fort Defiance	27	45,241
Tuba City	14	53,000
Newlands	5	5,995
Dilcon sub-office	5	6,743
Kayenta	7	15,000

JUSTIFICATION FOR FY 1995 FUNDING

PRIORITY: Funds to renovate the administration and/or clinic facilities of Chinle Agency.

AGENCY: Department of the Interior and Related Agencies
Department of Health & Human Service
Indian Health Service

FISCAL YEAR: 1995

APPROPRIATION: 0

ACTIVITY: These funds are requested to maintain the inhouse management and/or clinical operations of Chinle Agency which oversees the community health concerns of 15 chapters with an approximate population of 22,993 surrounding the agency.

PROPOSED REQUEST: $1,000,000
To be utilized for renovation costs of strengthening building structure, asbestos abatement, stabilizing foundation, lighting and heating fixtures and any proposed expansions to facilities.

CURRENT PROGRAM: The agency programs are currently under the operational costs of the Department of Behavioral Health which is a composite of the Division of Health which receives its sources from the Health Care Improvement Act, P.L. 94-437, the Indian Health Self-Determination Act P.L. 99-570, Navajo Nation General Funds, the Center for Substance Abuse Funds and some state funds.

AMOUNT BUDGETED IN FISCAL YEAR '95: 0

FEASIBILITY: All of these buildings in which the staff is housed and to where the clients go to receive their health care are decades old and have become dilapidated to the point of needing constant repair and are becoming unsafe and hazardous to both staff and clients by not meeting building safety standards. IHS, which provides for some repair costs at the agencies and sub-offices is finding it impossible to keep up with the rising costs of the maintenance of all agency facilities while trying to stabilize personal health care costs of its population.

JUSTIFICATION FOR FY 1995 FUNDING

PRIORITY: Funds to renovate the administration and/or clinic facilities of Shiprock Agency.

AGENCY: Department of the Interior and Related Agencies
Department of Health & Human Service
Indian Health Service

FISCAL YEAR: 1995

APPROPRIATION: 0

ACTIVITY: These funds are requested to maintain the inhouse management and/or clinical operations of Shiprock Agency which oversees the community health concerns of 21 chapters with an approximate population of 26,230 surrounding the agency.

PROPOSED REQUEST: **$1,000,000**
To be utilized for renovation costs of strengthening building structure, asbestos abatement, stabilizing foundation, lighting and heating fixtures and any proposed expansions to facilities.

CURRENT PROGRAM: The agency programs are currently under the operational costs of the Department of Behavioral Health which is a composite of the Division of Health which receives its sources from the Health Care Improvement Act, P.L. 94-437, the Indian Health Self-Determination Act P.L. 99-570, Navajo Nation General Funds, the Center for Substance Abuse Funds and some state funds.

AMOUNT BUDGETED IN FISCAL YEAR '95: 0

FEASIBILITY: All of these buildings in which the staff is housed and to where the clients go to receive their health care are decades old and have become dilapidated to the point of needing constant repair and are becoming unsafe and hazardous to both staff and clients by not meeting building safety standards. IHS, which provides for some repair costs at the agencies and sub-offices is finding it impossible to keep up with the rising costs of the maintenance of all agency facilities while trying to stabilize personal health care costs of its population.

JUSTIFICATION FOR FY 1995 FUNDING

PRIORITY: Funds to renovate the administration and/or clinic facilities of Crownpoint Agency.

AGENCY: Department of the Interior and Related Agencies
Department of Health & Human Service
Indian Health Service

FISCAL YEAR: 1995

APPROPRIATION: 0

ACTIVITY: These funds are requested to maintain the inhouse management and/or clinical operations of Crownpoint Agency which oversees the community health concerns of 31 chapters with an approximate population of 27,458 surrounding the agency.

PROPOSED REQUEST: **$1,000,000**
To be utilized for renovation costs of strengthening building structure, asbestos abatement, stabilizing foundation, lighting and heating fixtures and any proposed expansions to facilities.

CURRENT PROGRAM: The agency programs are currently under the operational costs of the Department of Behavioral Health which is a composite of the Division of Health which receives its sources from the Health Care Improvement Act, P.L. 94-437, the Indian Health Self-Determination Act P.L. 99-570, Navajo Nation General Funds, the Center for Substance Abuse Funds and some state funds.

AMOUNT BUDGETED IN FISCAL YEAR '95: 0

FEASIBILITY: All of these buildings in which the staff is housed and to where the clients go to receive their health care are decades old and have become dilapidated to the point of needing constant repair and are becoming unsafe and hazardous to both staff and clients by not meeting building safety standards. IHS, which provides for some repair costs at the agencies and sub-offices is finding it impossible to keep up with the rising costs of the maintenance of all agency facilities while trying to stabilize personal health care costs of its population.

JUSTIFICATION FOR FY 1995 FUNDING

PRIORITY: Funds to renovate the administration and/or clinic facilities of Fort Defiance Agency.

AGENCY: Department of the Interior and Related Agencies
Department of Health & Human Service
Indian Health Service

FISCAL YEAR: 1995

APPROPRIATION: 0

ACTIVITY: These funds are requested to maintain the inhouse management and/or clinical operations of Fort Defiance Agency which oversees the community health concerns of 27 chapters with an approximate population of 45,241 surrounding the agency.

PROPOSED REQUEST: $1,000,000
To be utilized for renovation costs of strengthening building structure, asbestos abatement, stabilizing foundation, lighting and heating fixtures and any proposed expansions to facilities.

CURRENT PROGRAM: The agency programs are currently under the operational costs of the Department of Behavioral Health which is a composite of the Division of Health which receives its sources from the Health Care Improvement Act, P.L. 94-437, the Indian Health Self-Determination Act P.L. 99-570, Navajo Nation General Funds, the Center for Substance Abuse Funds and some state funds.

AMOUNT BUDGETED IN FISCAL YEAR '95: 0

FEASIBILITY: All of these buildings in which the staff is housed and to where the clients go to receive their health care are decades old and have become dilapidated to the point of needing constant repair and are becoming unsafe and hazardous to both staff and clients by not meeting building safety standards. IHS, which provides for some repair costs at the agencies and sub-offices is finding it impossible to keep up with the rising costs of the maintenance of all agency facilities while trying to stabilize personal health care costs of its population.

JUSTIFICATION FOR FY 1995 FUNDING

PRIORITY: Funds to renovate the administration and/or clinic facilities of Newlands Agency.

AGENCY: Department of the Interior and Related Agencies
Department of Health & Human Service
Indian Health Service

FISCAL YEAR: 1995

APPROPRIATION: 0

ACTIVITY: These funds are requested to maintain the inhouse management and/or clinical operations of Newlands Agency which oversees the community health concerns of 5 chapters with an approximate population of 5,995 surrounding the agency.

PROPOSED REQUEST: $1,000,000
To be utilized for renovation costs of strengthening building structure, asbestos abatement, stabilizing foundation, lighting and heating fixtures and any proposed expansions to facilities.

CURRENT PROGRAM: The agency programs are currently under the operational costs of the Department of Behavioral Health which is a composite of the Division of Health which receives its sources from the Health Care Improvement Act, P.L. 94-437, the Indian Health Self-Determination Act P.L. 99-570, Navajo Nation General Funds, the Center for Substance Abuse Funds and some state funds.

AMOUNT BUDGETED IN FISCAL YEAR '95: 0

FEASIBILITY: All of these buildings in which the staff is housed and to where the clients go to receive their health care are decades old and have become dilapidated to the point of needing constant repair and are becoming unsafe and hazardous to both staff and clients by not meeting building safety standards. IHS, which provides for some repair costs at the agencies and sub-offices is finding it impossible to keep up with the rising costs of the maintenance of all agency facilities while trying to stabilize personal health care costs of its population.

JUSTIFICATION FOR FY 1995 FUNDING

PRIORITY: Funds to renovate the administration and/or clinic facilities of the Dilcon Sub-Office.

AGENCY: Department of the Interior and Related Agencies
Department of Health & Human Service
Indian Health Service

FISCAL YEAR: 1995

APPROPRIATION: 0

ACTIVITY: These funds are requested to maintain the inhouse management and/or clinical operations of the Dilcon Sub-Office which oversees the community health concerns of 5 chapters with an approximate population of 6,743 surrounding the agency.

PROPOSED REQUEST: $1,000,000
To be utilized for renovation costs of strengthening building structure, asbestos abatement, stabilizing foundation, lighting and heating fixtures and any proposed expansions to facilities.

CURRENT PROGRAM: The agency programs are currently under the operational costs of the Department of Behavioral Health which is a composite of the Division of Health which reCeives its sources from the Health Care Improvement Act, P.L. 94-437, the Indian Health Self-Determination Act P.L. 99-570, Navajo Nation General Funds, the Center for Substance Abuse Funds and some state funds.

AMOUNT BUDGETED IN FISCAL YEAR '95: 0

FEASIBILITY: All of these buildings in which the staff is housed and to where the clients go to receive their health care are decades old and have become dilapidated to the point of needing constant repair and are becoming unsafe and hazardous to both staff and clients by not meeting building safety standards. IHS, which provides for some repair costs at the agencies and sub-offices is finding it impossible to keep up with the rising costs of the maintenance of all agency facilities while trying to stabilize personal health care costs of its population.

JUSTIFICATION FOR FY 1995 FUNDING

PRIORITY: Funds to renovate the administration and/or clinic facilities of Tuba City Agency.

AGENCY: Department of the Interior and Related Agencies
Department of Health & Human Service
Indian Health Service

FISCAL YEAR: 1995

APPROPRIATION: 0

ACTIVITY: These funds are requested to maintain the inhouse management and/or clinical operations of Tuba City Agency which oversees the community health concerns of 14 chapters with an approximate population of 49,000 surrounding the agency.

PROPOSED REQUEST: $1,000,000
To be utilized for renovation costs of strengthening building structure, asbestos abatement, stabilizing foundation, lighting and heating fixtures and any proposed expansions to facilities.

CURRENT PROGRAM: The agency programs are currently under the operational costs of the Department of Behavioral Health which is a composite of the Division of Health which receives its sources from the Health Care Improvement Act, P.L. 94-437, the Indian Health Self-Determination Act P.L. 99-570, Navajo Nation General Funds, the Center for Substance Abuse Funds and some state funds.

AMOUNT BUDGETED IN FISCAL YEAR '95: 0

FEASIBILITY: All of these buildings in which the staff is housed and to where the clients go to receive their health care are decades old and have become dilapidated to the point of needing constant repair and are becoming unsafe and hazardous to both staff and clients by not meeting building safety standards. IHS, which provides for some repair costs at the agencies and sub-offices is finding it impossible to keep up with the rising costs of the maintenance of all agency facilities while trying to stabilize personal health care costs of its population.

JUSTIFICATION FOR FY 1995 FUNDING

PRIORITY: Funds to renovate the administration and/or clinic facilities of Kayenta Agency.

AGENCY: Department of the Interior and Related Agencies
Department of Health & Human Service
Indian Health Service

FISCAL YEAR: 1995

APPROPRIATION: 0

ACTIVITY: These funds are requested to maintain the inhouse management and/or clinical operations of Kayenta Agency which oversees the community health concerns of 7 chapters with an approximate population of 15,000 surrounding the agency.

PROPOSED REQUEST: $1,000,000
To be utilized for renovation costs of strengthening building structure, asbestos abatement, stabilizing foundation, lighting and heating fixtures and any proposed expansions to facilities.

CURRENT PROGRAM: The agency programs are currently under the operational costs of the Department of Behavioral Health which is a composite of the Division of Health which receives its sources from the Health Care Improvement Act, P.L. 94-437, the Indian Health Self-Determination Act P.L. 99-570, Navajo Nation General Funds, the Center for Substance Abuse Funds and some state funds.

AMOUNT BUDGETED IN FISCAL YEAR '95: 0

FEASIBILITY: All of these buildings in which the staff is housed and to where the clients go to receive their health care are decades old and have become dilapidated to the point of needing constant repair and are becoming unsafe and hazardous to both staff and clients by not meeting building safety standards. IHS, which provides for some repair costs at the agencies and sub-offices is finding it impossible to keep up with the rising costs of the maintenance of all agency facilities while trying to stabilize personal health care costs of its population.

EXHIBIT "F"

A COMPREHENSIVE MENTAL HEALTH CARE SYSTEM FOR NATIVE AMERICANS IN NEW MEXICO

A Report of the Native American Mental Health Planning Project

EXECUTIVE SUMMARY

November, 1993

University of New Mexico
Department of Psychiatry
Center on Alcoholism, Substance Abuse, and Addictions (CASAA)

Authors:

Philip A. May, Ph.D., Principal Investigator
Maria G. Chavez
Jan P. Gossage, M.A.
Diane LeResche, Ph.D.
Joe Neidhardt, M.D.
Mary Roessel, M.D.
Delores D. Stroud, M.B.A.
Nadine Tafoya, M.S.W.
Alice R. Velarde, M.S.W.

Funded in part by:
The State Department of Health
Mental Health Division
Contract No. 93.665.62.351

A COMPREHENSIVE MENTAL HEALTH CARE SYSTEM FOR NATIVE AMERICANS* IN NEW MEXICO

EXECUTIVE SUMMARY

This is a summary of the November, 1993 report of the Native American Mental Health Planning Project for the state of New Mexico. The report is the product of a seven-month contract from the State Division of Mental Health to the University of New Mexico, Department of Psychiatry/Center on Alcoholism, Substance Abuse, and Addictions (CASAA) and the planning efforts that it stimulated. A Select Committee of representatives from New Mexico tribes, appropriate state and federal agencies, private entities, and consumers have provided input throughout the planning process. The bulk of the organizing, planning, and writing has been carried out by an interdisciplinary team of employees of the University of New Mexico, consultants from a variety of agencies including the Indian Health Service (IHS), the Bureau of Indian Affairs (BIA), and others. Only a portion of this overall effort was financed by the State contract with other contributions of time and effort coming from many individuals and agencies. In 1992, prior to the planning process, letters of support for the project were obtained from all tribal leaders in the state.

Based upon the findings of this planning effort, a system of comprehensive mental health care for American Indians is proposed. This continuum of care extends from the tribal

* The terms Native American, Native, and American Indian are used synonymously in this summary and report.

communities, to regional centers of care, to a centralized facility. The regional and central facilities exist for highly specialized care which cannot be adequately carried out in local communities.

Methodology

The final plan is based on the collection and triangulation of a variety of types of information and data characterizing the need for mental health services and concepts of how to best provide the highest quality of care for Native Americans of all ages in the State of New Mexico. The primary sources utilized in the document are:

- a review of the existing literature on American Indian health and mental health, plans, and needs assessments on Indian mental health;
- an indirect measure of the magnitude of alcohol, drug abuse, and mental health needs using selected measures from current census data;
- an extensive survey of current agencies providing services;
- a clinical programming survey to select from optional mental health care delivery system models and a prioritization of services needed;
- the ideas, visions, suggestions, and recommendations of the Select Committee and its subcommittees; and
- private interviews and focus group discussions with tribal members, service workers, and tribal leaders.

Findings from the Literature Review

American Indians represent 8.9% of the population of New Mexico. New Mexico has the fourth greatest number of Native Americans and the second largest percentage of any state. The

Indian population of the State is the fastest growing ethnic group and by the time the ten-year planning/construction/ implementation phases of this report are completed (2003) there will be 181,379 Indians in the State. This is a 35% increase. Therefore, estimates of need many also increase by a similar factor.

The Native American population in New Mexico is primarily a young one with a lower proportion of males than any other ethnic group. Therefore, the health, mental health, and substance abuse problems predominant among most tribal communities are those of younger individuals. American Indian males suffer substantially higher rates of violent death than other groups in New Mexico. Such causes which are usually classified as parapsychiatric in nature include: motor vehicle crashes, other injuries, suicide, homicide, and other substance and alcohol-related problems such as cirrhosis of the liver, alcohol dependence syndrome, and alcoholic psychosis. This is in spite of the fact that a lower percentage of adult New Mexico Indians drink than do adults of most other groups in the nation and the state. The generation of such high rates of substance abuse-related death stems from a higher proportion of heavy and abusive drinkers among those Indian adolescents and adults who do drink. Fetal Alcohol Syndrome has become a problem among New Mexico Indians in the past 15 years, and it is, on average, twice as high among New Mexico Indians as among other people in the U.S. There is extreme variation in all of the above problems from one tribal community to the next. Some Indian communities have few problems while others have a substantial prevalence of them.

The literature review yielded many studies relevant to American Indian mental health in the areas of: epidemiology (prevalence patterns, and overall causes of problems), individual mental health disturbances treated in clinics, and issues and models of service delivery. In some other states and in Canada, studies have shown that substantial mental health and substance abuse needs were present in Indian communities. In various Indian community studies, the range of those found to be in definite need of psychiatric and mental health services ranged from 25% in Oklahoma, to 37% in Northern Canada, to 54% in a northwest coastal community. Overall, various research efforts have broken the estimates of problems and need into severe or substantial problems, moderate to mild, minimal, and none. Generally community surveys and treated prevalence studies consistently implicated alcohol abuse-related problems and disorders, depression, anxiety, and transient disturbances as the leading mental health problems found in Native communities throughout the continent. An increasing concern about domestic violence, child abuse and neglect, and other forms of multi-problem family behavior has also emerged in the extant literature.

Regional studies in the Southwest are generally supportive of the above conclusions. Problem drinking indicators, depression, anxiety, marital problems, and situational disturbances are also the most commonly treated problems in both health and mental health clinics and hospitals serving American Indians in New Mexico. In one recent study alcohol problems accounted for 75% of inpatient mental health episodes at New

Mexico IHS and contract hospitals and 52% of the Indian Health Service (IHS) outpatient episodes. Overall, 21% of New Mexico Indians of all ages will utilize an IHS facility for a mental health/substance abuse problem over a ten-year period. This, therefore, is a measure of treated prevalence. New Mexico Indian studies also indicate that child abuse and neglect are problems which are most commonly alcohol related, but alcohol abuse is not a singular cause of abuse and neglect or of any of these problems.

There has been a number of comprehensive studies and reviews of American Indian mental health dating back as far as 1969. The literature review highlights fifteen major studies, books, reports, and/or mental health system plans which have been published over the past 24 years. Most of these studies and plans are very comprehensive but most importantly very consistent in their findings and recommendations. The most common problems and concepts which emerge repeatedly are: alcohol abuse and its sequelae, family disruption, suicide, depression; there is a real need for cultural sensitivity; there exists a need to train and utilize indigenous workers; and there exist a number of major barriers to mental health care.

Highlighted in the literature review of the report are a number of "ideal" or "model" programs known to the project planning staff. Furthermore, the most useful and carefully prepared results of the other extant planning documents are summarized. In general it becomes evident from the literature review that we in New Mexico are not the first to "walk this path" or "plow this ground." What we might be first in doing, a need for increased cultural sensitivity to be used in mental health care, a need for increasing Indian access to care, and a need for training more Indian mental health professionals.

Inpatient utilization data from IHS hospitals and contract care in New Mexico are also summariezed in the report. Confirmation of the importance of alcohol abuse problems was evident. Since IHS admissions, particularly in contract hospitals, are limited by space, dollars, and other available resources, these treated prevalence data represent a highly restricted characterization of need. Examining only these data, one gets the impression that utilization (and therefore need?) is quite low. Other indicators, however, tell a different story about magniture of need.

Vision statements produced by members of the Project Select Committee provided the basis for the initial needs surveys and for the eventual planning of service delivery models. A number of these visions are depicted in full in the report. A summary of the common themes and concepts is also reported. Additionally the visions of the Select Committee led to the development of four prototype models which were then sent out to mental health professionals and tribal leaders throughout the state along with programming and service delivery questionnaires. The results of this assessment and the vision statements were then carefully translated into the system design.

Finally, stakeholder interviews and focus groups of tribal and communities leaders and consumers were used to further define local concerns, issues, and ideas. Special tribal cultural traits and community desires were assessed for further definition of appropriate needs and services.

Guiding Principles

Mental illness in this report has been viewed in the broadest possible perspective. The planning has been pursued from a comprehensive behavioral health approach which includes both psychiatric and parapsychiatric problems. Substance abuse, child abuse and neglect, multiple diagnosis and dual diagnosis problems, neurological disorders, and other behavioral health issues commonly of concern in Indian communities were all included in the planning. A holistic approach is used. The holistic approach encompasses the mind, the body, and the spiritual. The fact that each Native American tribe in New Mexico has its own holistic perspective was carefully considered, and the plan attempts to embrace services and approaches which allow for the specific application of traditional tribal views within their communities and the total system.

The mental health system for Native Americans that is proposed will have a comprehensive network of services for the prevention, intervention, and treatment of mild and serious behavioral health problems. Both minor problems and serious mental illnesses are addressed for people of all ages. Personnel, facilities, services, and other dimensions of the system will be culturally sensitive and appropriate. The goal is to enable all people to be well-integrated members of their family, extended family, and community. The maintaining and restoration of harmony and balance within community systems is vital to the accomplishment of this goal. Treatments will meet the unique needs of the individual and of his/her Native American community. Services must be accessible in all respects: geographically, financially, culturally, and temporally. Services will be provided in the least restrictive environment possible given the presenting problem. Confidentiality will be maintained throughout the system via principles, technology, and policy.

All levels of care are proposed in the plan:

- some crisis response capability will exist in each community;
- thorough evaluations of most mental health problems will be available at one of a variety of locales;
- a comprehensive variety of treatment modalities utilizing the strengths of both traditional American Indian cultures and western medical care are provided;
- coordinated relationships with all health and social services agencies are facilitated; and
- extensive follow through care in the local and regional levels is the goal for both referral and aftercare.

Local, community-based care and services are always emphasized. Cooperation among spiritual, medical, and psychosocial healers will occur, along with the integration of the strengths of the extended family and community. Joint Commission on Accreditation of Health Care Organizations (JCAHO) or equivalent standards will be met.

Basic Design of the Proposed System

Three levels of care are proposed in the system, with personnel, transportation, and computer links between them providing for a complete continuum of support and care. These levels provide services at community, regional, and central locations. The majority of the care will be primary care (basic supportive care) delivered in the local communities. The regional and central care levels will provide secondary and tertiary services, and will be supportive and readily available, yet the centralized levels will account for a minority percentage of the total activity (See Diagram A).

Community-based, outpatient family and client-centered services are envisioned as the most comprehensive and important component of this system. Each community will have a Community Service Guide and a Community Response Team. These people will oversee all mental health services for the local, tribal community through planning, provision of services, and coordination. They will also work jointly to provide for a variety of services in the community, from various types of prevention and recommendations for public policy to the primary care of mental health problems. Support services of all kinds such as mental health education, social work, outpatient psychiatric care, outpatient alcohol treatment and substance abuse prevention services, and other services are provided at this level (See Diagram B). Interactive and cooperative care with all local community resources and mental health services is mandated at this level. This includes coordination with traditional healers and traditional ceremonies and medicine as appropriate for each tribe.

The plan also calls for five regional facilities, optimally located on tribal land throughout the state. At the regional centers, secondary care will be delivered for more challenging and complex problems. Each of these facilities will have a day

Diagram A

Overall Program Design

The program will provide primary care at the community level, secondary care at satellite facilities, and tertiary care at the central location. Both the satellite and central facility will provide support for community programs. The emphasis will be to treat the individual within the context of the family in the community whenever possible.

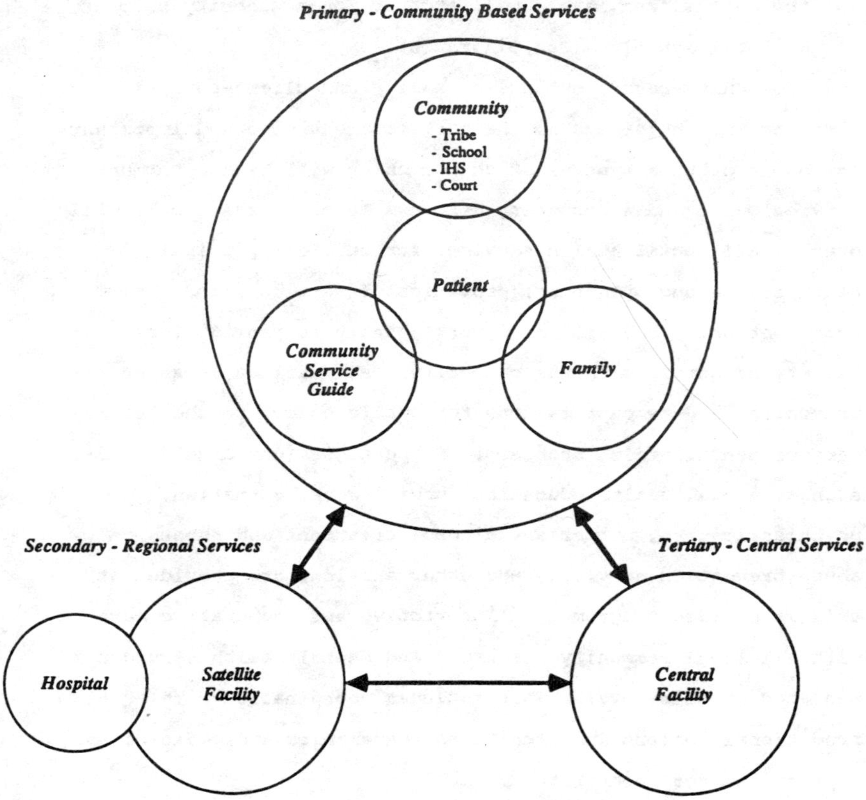

Diagram B

Community Response Team

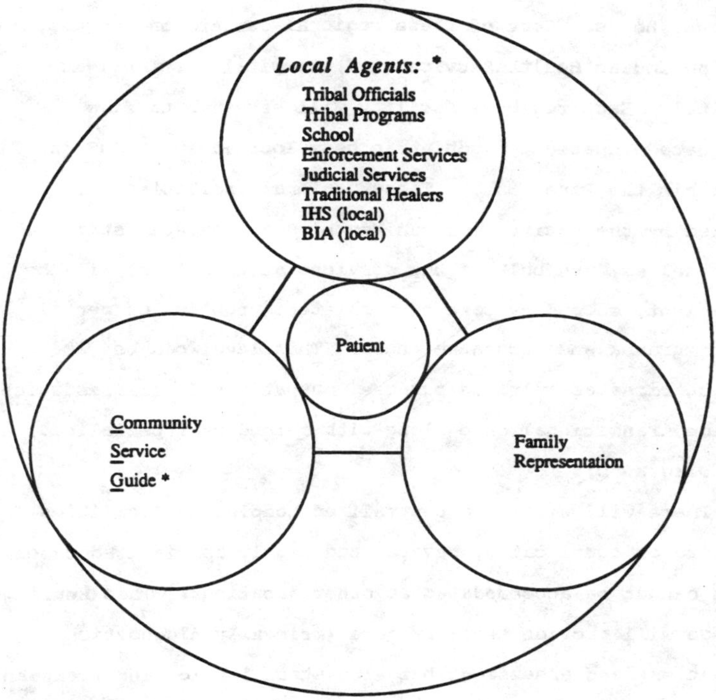

* The Community Response Team is united in a comprehensive regional network of communication which is linked externally with the other levels of the Native American Mental Health System.

treatment center (Pine House) and care managers (See Diagram C). The size and cultural orientation of the programs will depend on the regional location, the tribal culture of the area, and regional needs. Some of these regional centers may be associated with an Indian Health Service (IHS) hospital, or a private hospital. Each regional facility will have two to five designated inpatient psychiatric beds located in an IHS facility or within the Pine House. These regional facilities will be staffed by the Native American Mental Health System staff. Nevertheless, the bulk of the services at this level will be outpatient, secondary care of persistent problems of mental health trauma and substance abuse. This level can be characterized as multiple purpose, outpatient facilities which provide transitional care along with secondary (specialized) care (See Diagram D).

There will also be a centralized complex of facilities for the care of complicated, severe, and highly specialized cases which cannot be accommodated at other locations. This Healing Village will provide tertiary care (primarily diagnostic evaluations and assessment but also stabilization and treatment) for difficult cases. The goal of this centralized complex will be to develop treatment plans and protocols, in conjunction with the regional and community staff, which can then be carried out in the regional or local sites once the diagnosis is made and the patient stabilized. The Healing Village will consist of: a Welcome House for extensive evaluations; three Peaceful Homes with a total of 24 beds for acute, short-term inpatient treatment (one home of 8 beds each for children, adolescents, and adults);

Diagram C

Satellite Regional Facility - Secondary Services

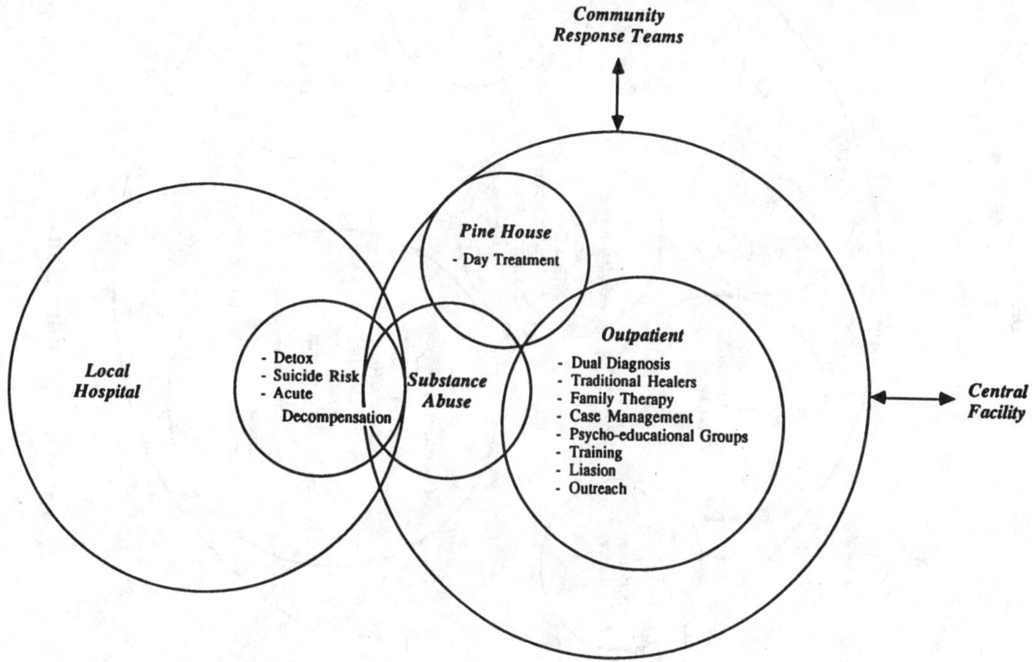

Diagram D

Regional Facility Detail

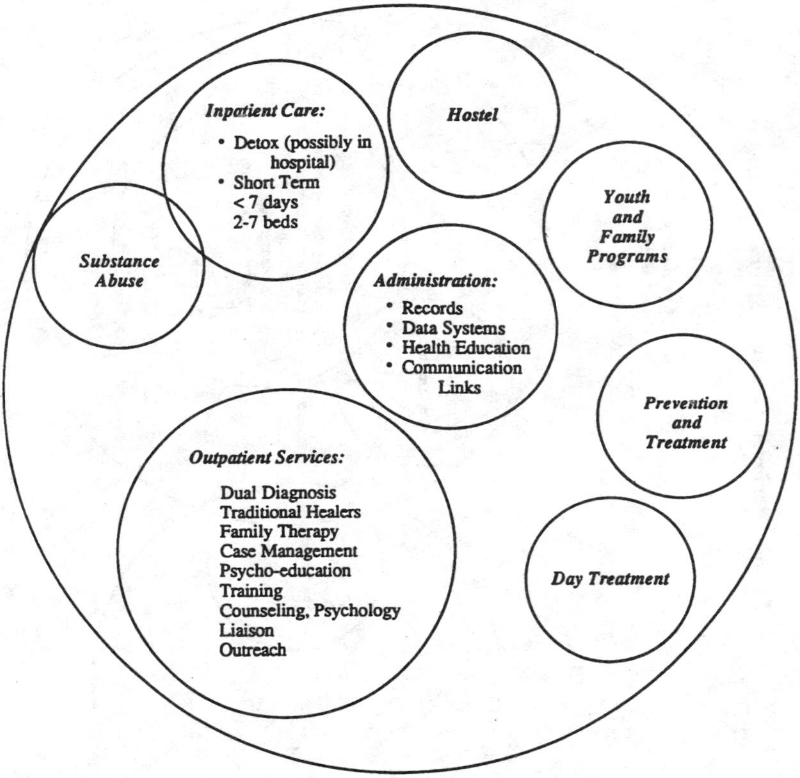

Pine House

a home for outpatient day treatment (Big Pine House); and short-term living areas (called the Share and Care Hostel) for families and local healers and support staff involved in a patient's treatment and discharge planning (See Diagram E). There will also be health education offices, administrative offices, and a computerized client management information system located at the central site. These services will connect with the regional and local sites. In addition to providing treatment services for clients, this facility will provide training and technical assistance to all communities and service providers.

Native healing and a variety of religious practices (Native traditional, Christian, and others) are seen as integral to this system, as they contribute greatly to the holistic approach. In the planning, however, it was clear that there are different perceptions as to how traditional medicine and religious practices are to be integrated. While the Navajo spokespersons were very enthusiastic about the full participation of Navajo healers and the integration of Navajo medicine principals in all levels of the system, the Pueblo spokespersons took the opposite view. Pueblo religion and medicine must be kept separate from the system and should only be sought rather independently on a case-by-case basis by the families and individuals involved. The Apache spokespersons generally concurred with the Pueblo stance. Therefore, the system and its personnel can and should integrate specific Native healing only to the extent desired by particular tribes and individuals, but must be open to integrate whenever desired, desirable, and possible. The system and its personnel must be culturally aware and sensitive at all times.

Diagram E

The Healing Village
Tertiary Site

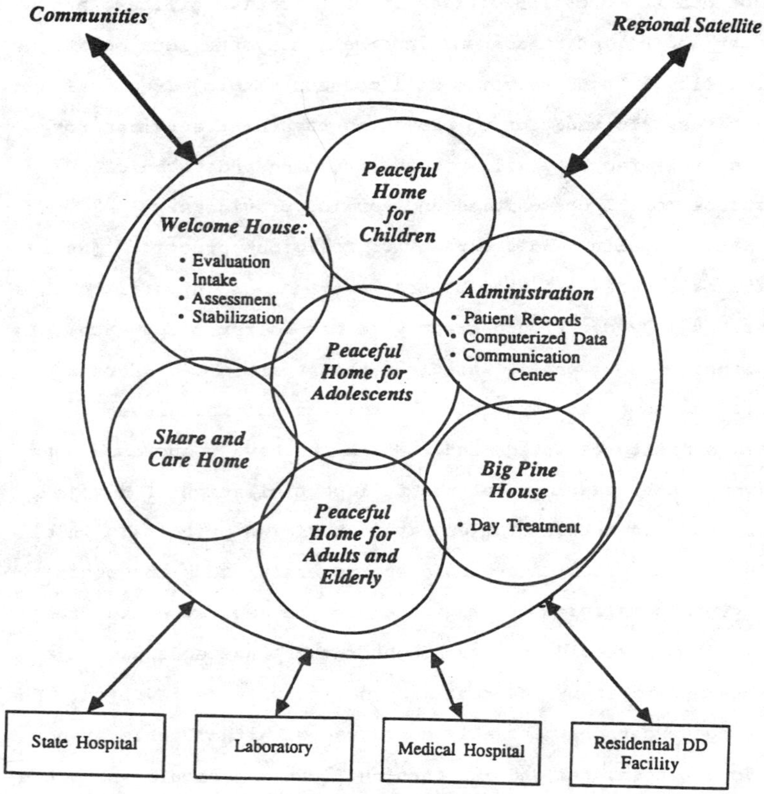

Facilities at all levels are to mirror, and be sensitive to, the cultural groups they serve. They are to provide a Native, home-like atmosphere. Architectural design and development teams should have well-established track records of working with and on Native projects and in consulting tribal members in the design process. Similarly, the service providers at all levels will be those individuals who are professionally competent, bi-cultural and/or culturally sensitive, and who can mesh interaction, diagnoses, treatment, and family/patient education to the tribal and cultural traditions of New Mexico Indians.

Structure and Organization of the System

A not-for-profit organization might be established. Programs and facilities are to be governed, administered, managed, and developed by New Mexico tribal members.

Initially, a temporary consortium which is representative of all the New Mexico tribes might be brought together, primarily to structure and select members of the first Central Governing Council. The Consortium should have representatives appointed by the heads of the following tribes, bands, chapters, and groups: Each of the 19 Pueblos; the Jicarilla Apache; Mescalero Apache; Cañoncito, Alamo, and Ramah Navajo reservations; Gallup, Crownpoint, and Shiprock Navajo areas of the main Navajo reservation; and urban Indians. Representatives of Native American consumers and families should be included in the above delegates. Traditional healers might also be represented where tribal culture permits.

The Central Council will oversee the implementation of the

system. It will have the overall responsibility for setting policy to establish and maintain the complete continuum of care. Each site (main and regional) should have an Advisory Council, consisting of local members selected by the tribes it serves (See Diagram I). These Advisory Councils will interact with the local Community Response Teams and local units of government.

Funding Considerations

The continuum of care might be accomplished without any new construction. By utilizing existing and renovated facilities, the continuum of care might be established quickly and for a reasonable cost. As noted in the report, a number of IHS general medical facilities are under-utilized and might be reprogrammed and reconfigured for full participation in this system of comprehensive care.

Estimates of new construction were obtained by the project. An estimate for the cost of the new construction of the facilities and the equipment proposed at the Healing Village is $19 million (137,000 sq. ft.). A rough estimate of the cost of new construction and equipment for the regional Pine Houses is $1.1 million (10,000 sq. ft.) each. Both of these estimates assumes spacious, culturally appropriate designs. It does not include the potential cost of lands, nor the option of renovating existing buildings. Estimates of operating expenses for the system are computed and contained in the larger report. These calculations were produced in collaboration with the Albuquerque Area BIA Facilities Planning Office.

Potential funders for the continuum of care have not yet

Diagram I

Governing Organization/Structure of the Native American Mental Health System

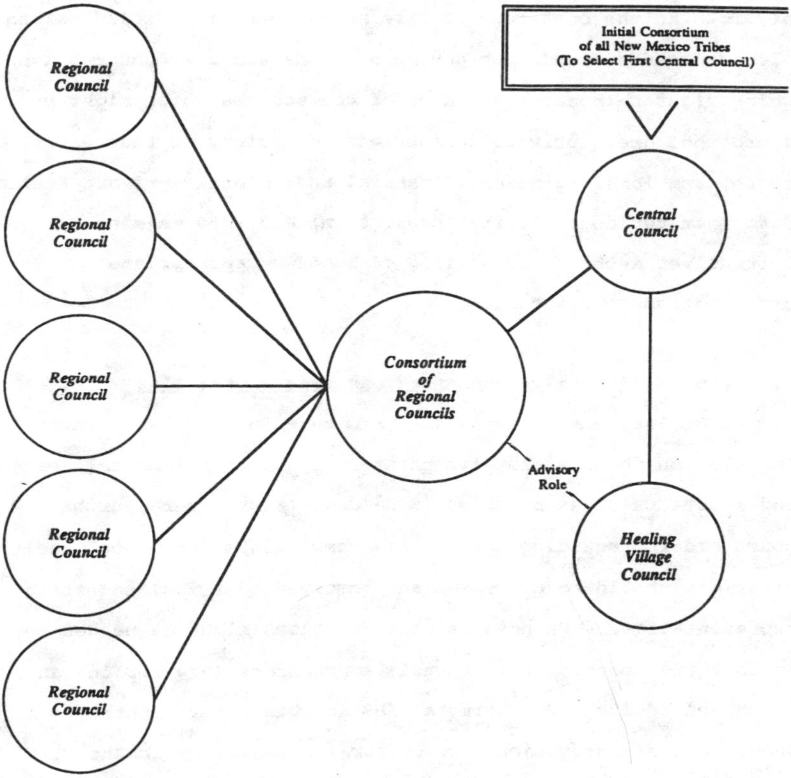

been identified or approached. Some of the continuum of care is already in place in the form of services provided by IHS, BIA, tribes and the state. These existing services could be woven from existing funding sources. Funding for new items and services in the continuum of care needs to be identified, along with sources of funds for any renovations and new construction which might be necessary. Some of the sources which might be approached are: private foundations; a variety of federal, state, and local agencies; financial and/or other private health care institutions; a tribal consortium; and fund raising initiatives such as the selling of bonds by appropriate organizations and agencies.

6. **Some Additional Recommendations Made in the Plan**

Legislative recommendations are made in the plan. State legislation which would give partnership to tribal mental health and substance abuse programs is needed. Furthermore, tribal court orders regarding involuntary commitments for mental health treatment should be discussed and resolved by tribal and state representatives. Changes in state statutes might be needed to support the concept of culturally appropriate care for Indian youth and adults. Furthermore, IHS inpatient care contracts should contain provisions for cultural sensitivity in the provision of care. Policies and legislative provisions are needed to provide public and private recognition and benefits for traditional Native American healing practices as defined to be appropriate by each tribe.

Consideration should also be given to changing tribal codes

which do not yet address mental health issues. Tribes can empower themselves greatly with such codes.

Personnel issues are also central to the plan. There is a shortage of trained Native Americans, and others sensitive to Native American mental health issues, to meet the personnel needs of this system. Educational institutions and programs in New Mexico should be encouraged to work to meet the personnel needs through recruitment of students to existing programs and the creation of new credential programs and continuing education curricula relevant to Native American mental health.

A ten-year time frame is the last part of the project report. It is not unreasonable that this entire system can be in place and functioning in a matter of six to seven years and fully solidified at the end of ten years. Details are presented.

EXHIBIT "G"

DEPARTMENT OF HEALTH & HUMAN SERVICES

Public Health Service
Health Services Administration

24 Mar 94

Navajo Area
Indian Health Service
Tuba City Indian Medical Center
Tuba City, Arizona 86045

Norman Ration
Director, Department of Behavioral Health Services
The Navajo Nation
PO Box 709
Window Rock, AZ 86515

MAR 31 1994

Dear Mr. Ration,

I am writing in response to your request of this morning for a summary of the services provided and needed in the area of Mental Health on the Navajo reservation. Obviously, this has never been a wealthy program, and so the thought of "tightening our belts" in the spirit of government "reinvention", while appealing in the abstract, is actually an insult to the intelligence of anyone truly aware of the conditions faced by our mentally ill or alcoholic community members.

Currently there are excellent resources available through Navajo Area IHS for people in need of short-term outpatient care for acute mental health problems of mild to moderate severity. There is also outpatient substance abuse counseling avalable through your program. Unfortunately, the people most in need of our services - those with severe mental illnesses, those in need of residential alcohol rehab, and children in need of long-term treatment and supervision - are already poorly served in most cases

There is no day treatment of any kind for severely mentally ill Navajo adults anywhere on the reservation except for Kayenta , where the program has received one-time one-year funding through IHS Contract Health 'left over' dollars from the end of fiscal year 1993. This program has already demonstrated major savings in the form of prevention of re-hospitalization for the patients receiving these services.

There is no clear avenue for the funding of long-term placement of children who, because of risky behavior (chronic suicidality, perpetration of sexual offenses, running away, drug abuse, truancy, etc.) require a placement more intensive than a foster or group home for an extended period of time. This is particularly true for the increasing number of children affected by Fetal Alcohol Syndrome with its associated impulsive behavior, poor social adjustment, and risk of substance abuse. Without the employment of long-term specialized rehab modalities, these children are likely to end up in the criminal justice system. In addition, the foster-care program on the reservation is overburdened to the breaking point. There are not enough foster homes, those families willing to provide homes are not trained or supported adequately due to a shortage of resources, and there are no therapeutic foster homes at all

Finally, the problems of alcoholism - medical, vocational, social, community, and in multi-generational and cultural self-esteem - are not being addressed as a high priority despite political claims to the contrary. For example, our community tries to encourage involvement of fathers in their children's lives and prosecutes for non-payment of child support and yet, should that adult male present himself in need of alcohol rehab, he will usually be told at our DBHS agency that there are no resources for his treatment.... although an adolescent or a woman does receive special funding - through "fad" interests of the congress in FAS prevention or the like. There is not a single comprehensive adult alcohol rehabilitation facility with available medical services anywhere on this reservation, the largest in the United States. This should be an embarrassment to the IHS, the federal government, and the tribe. It certainly is to many of us.

There is also no available inpatient psychiatric service for adults or children on the Navajo Reservation. People needing this care are transported far from their homes and families to expensive, for-profit facilities where often no staff member even speaks Navajo.

Money could be saved here; probably quite a bit - by developing cost-effective services close to home for our sickest patients with the most expensive problems, and recouping the Contract Health dollars saved. Reducing staff in existing facilities already overburdened (for example, the next appointment I have available is in three and a half weeks) would simply and definitely result in a decrease in the number of patients served and in the quality of their care. It would be great if there were fat to cut here. I would invite the senators and the President to visit the trailers and ramshackle buildings we do business out of before deciding we can absorb a 14% FTE reduction using creative "reinvention".

This is brief but I hope useful to you in your efforts. Please let me know if I can provide any further information.

Sincerely,

Elise Egerter, MD
Director of Mental Health
Tuba City Indian Medical Center

EE:ee

cc: T. Dudley Beck, MD
Abe Plummer, NAIHS Branch Chief
Frank Armao, MD, Area Clinical Consultant
Eva Smith, MD, Chief Clinical Consultant, Substance Abuse Branch, Hdq. West

EXHIBIT "H"

PROPOSAL

PREVALENCE OF ALCOHOL ABUSE AMONG THE NAVAJO

Submitted by:
Philip A. May, Ph.D., Director
Center on Alcoholism, Substance Abuse and Addictions
University of New Mexico
2350 Alamo S.E.
Albuquerque, New Mexico 87106
(505) 768-0107

Prepared: April 14, 1992

Introduction

The prevalence of substance abuse among adults, particularly alcohol use and abuse, has not been well studied among many American Indian tribes or groups of Alaska Natives. As of 1989, only six published articles had reached print in major academic journals or books (see May, 1989a). Certainly other studies have been done on alcohol use among Indian adults in other sites, but the data are not readily available nor easily accessible. Further, since tribes differ considerably from one another on a variety of behaviors, a study done on one reservation might not be too useful to another reservation or, even less useful to another tribe. Of the six published studies which involve Indian adults, two were done on the Standing Rock Sioux, two on the Navajo (main reservation), one on the Southern Ute and one on the Brokenhead Ojibway (in Canada). Most of these studies have used different criteria, the sample methods differ, the results were reported in different ways, and the time periods are very different (ranging from 1960 to 1984). Further, from a few unpublished health surveys, undertaken by the Indian Health Service in areas such as Aberdeen, some additional prevalence data might be available. Nevertheless, with the exception of the two studies on the Navajo, there are few prevalence data available for Navajo or Indian Adults which could be used to plan specific and targeted prevention or intervention programs for the Navajo Nation.

There have been a number of studies done on American Indian and Navajo school children. These studies, and their results, are available in a variety of publications (see May, 1989a and 1982 for references). Further, unpublished data and reports might be located in a number of agencies and states including New Mexico (May,1989b). Researchers such as Oetting and Beauvais (1985), Winfree and Griffiths (1983) and a number of tribes and agencies have done a considerable amount of surveying in this category. Further, these surveys have been put to use in creating school-based prevention programs in a variety of ways and in a variety of sites. Therefore, the prevalence of substance use and abuse among Indian school children is hardly an unstudied area, at least as far as surveys are concerned. It is the adult and non-school youth (dropout) prevalence and patterns about which we know the least, or have the least data.

The two published studies done among the Navajo were done by Levy and Kunitz (1974) and May and Smith (1988). In their book, Indian Drinking, Levy and Kunitz reported on studies done in 1969 among Navajos in four settings (two reservation areas, Flagstaff and a hospital sample). They found that 30% of Navajos who were 18 years old or older drink at least once a year. Males were considerably more likely to drink than were Navajo females (52% versus. 13%). May and Smith did a stratified sample at the Winslow I.H.S. Clinic in 1984 and found higher prevalence than the earlier Levy and Kunitz study; 52% of the Navajos sixteen years or older drank at least once a year (males = 64%, females = 40%). Therefore, the use of alcohol may be on the increase among the Navajo, particularly among females. Neither of these prevalence figures, however, are as high as the prevalence for the general U.S. But both studies, however, found that there were a substantial number of very heavy alcohol users within the Navajo drinker population, and that this proportion of problem drinkers was two to three times as great as among the general U.S. studies. None of the heaviest drinking alcohol abusers and alcoholics could be accessed in school studies.

Most studies which have tried to address the epidemiological features of Indian and Navajo drinking have done so by using indirect measures. Measures of mortality, morbidity, arrest, and protective custody are commonly used to measure the magnitude and nature of the problem. But these are not the best measures of true prevalence and incidence. They are merely outcome measures, generated to a substantial degree by the problem drinking segment of the population; and they tell us little about the nature of the drinking patterns of the overall Navajo population. Further, with the exception of the mortality measures, these data are in most cases duplicative counts. That is, one person can generate many episodes of illness, arrest and protective custody, and the data make it appear as if a large number of individuals have the same problem when in fact it may be a real minority of the Navajo population at any one time. Many beliefs supporting the "Drunken Indian Stereotype" and inadequate prevention programs are often perpetuated because of poor prevalence data, incomplete knowledge and inaccurate information (see May, 1989a). A prevalence study will define the accuracy of a variety of beliefs.

Therefore, a prevalence of drinking survey among a particular tribe is a rare and promising study. Such a survey among the adult population will allow a tribe: to identify the true extent of the problem, locate the traits and types of individuals who are at greatest risk for alcohol abuse, and to plan very specific and targeted treatment and prevention programs which are most appropriate for their people. Such a study should be of tremendous utility for the future.

Study Characteristics

The University of New Mexico, Center on Alcoholism, Substance Abuse and Addictions (CASAA), proposes to plan, organize and assist the Navajo Tribe, Department of Behavioral Health Services, in a study of the prevalence of Alcohol and Substance among its adult population. The study will have the following characteristics.

1. It will utilize a simple, random sample drawn from current tribal roles.

2. The study will focus on all Navajos enrolled and living on and adjacent to the reservation who are seventeen years of age or older. Special school samples will not be collected in this effort, for the emphasis is on the general Navajo adult population. If a person is a student, over sixteen, and is selected to be a participant in the study, then he/she will be included. Otherwise, neither students nor school samples will be included.

3. With the use of random sampling from the tribal roles, some of the sample will be drawn from all parts of the reservation in Arizona, New Mexico and Utah. Further, some data will be collected from Navajos living in border towns adjacent to the reservation and in the checkerboard area. Random methods should assure that a representative sample of persons from each agency will be drawn from tribal roles, but if necessary, representative proportions from the five agencies could be drawn. The questionnaire will document the agency of residence, so that the agency and area profiles might be constructed.

4. The simple, random sample method is deemed the most feasible and chosen as the sampling method of preference because it will allow for the most accurate information from a scientific point of view with the smallest possible sample. The I.H.S. estimated service population of the Navajo Area is 190,946. It is estimated that approximately 105,000 Navajo people will be in the 17+ ages (the median age of the tribe was found to be 19.9 years in 1990). The sample size that we propose to draw will be approximately 1,152. Based on random variation, this should provide a very representative sample from which the population characteristics can be determined. If 20 interviewers are utilized, each will have to do approximately 58 interviews, or if 15 interviewers are used, each will have to do 77 interviews.

5. The above sample size is calculated from standard mathematical formula on the selection of samples from relatively large populations. The formula used is as follows:

$$n = \frac{Np(1-p)}{(N-1)D + p(1-p)}$$

Where: N = population of the tribe; n = sample size: p = estimated true proportion of drinkers based on previous studies of the Navajo and tribes with similar levels of traditional social integration (see May, 1982 and 1989); and $D = e^2$ divided by four where e = maximal error. This provides a sample size calculation where the size of the population is known. The factor $p(1 - p)$ is maximum when $p = .50$ as might be expected among the Navajo. Using $p = .50$ yields the largest number of people who should be surveyed for the certainty of a minimal amount of error.

Using the above formula with a population the size of the Navajo, accuracy is ensured within 5 percentage points of true prevalence, and a confidence of 95%, with a sample size of 384. The sample of 1,152, therefore, will greatly improve on the above estimates of accuracy and should produce a sample with accuracy and confidence of the highest order possible.

6. The data will be collected orally by Navajo interviewers. The interviewers will be trained in a one to two day session on research project skills. The training will be done by U.N.M. Faculty and Navajo consultants at a workshop which can be held either on or adjacent to the Reservation.

Emphasized in the workshop will be: 1.) Interviewing skills, the purpose of the study, some scientific method and other technical issues. 2.) And translation, cultural issues in research, and confidentiality issues regarding the study.

7. The questionnaires will be set up so that they: are culturally sensitive and appropriate, can be given in either Navajo or English, and will yield data which are reliable, valid and can be compared to other studies of drinking prevalence, particularly national surveys. Therefore, questions will be asked in ways which will yield data which are similar to other surveys, but also will have questions of particular interest to the Navajo people. Most of the questions will be designed to delineate the epidemiology of alcohol and substance abuse and they will be directed a practical prevention and intervention needs. Also included will be several questions to elicit Navajo perceptions of the causes of, and the solutions to, the problem of alcohol and substance abuse. The total length of the questionnaire should not exceed ten pages. This will limit the respondent burden to no more than one-half hour, yet sufficient and valuable information will be collected.

8. The questionnaire will be prepared in cooperation, and with the input of, the Behavioral Health Services personnel. This should ensure the cultural relevancy of the various items picked, used or developed. Final discussions regarding the content of the questionnaire will be done in a meeting of representatives of both U.N.M. - C.A.S.A.A. and the Behavioral Health Services Division. After this meeting the questionnaire will be finalized, set up for computerization, and printed.

9. The data will be gathered by Behavioral Health Services staff. The interviews will be done in privacy at either the person's home, work or other appropriate location. Some interviews could be done by phone if deemed appropriate by both the Behavioral Health Services staff and the UNM researchers. The part of the sample for which the use of the phone is appropriate will have to be carefully considered, however. If the person chosen to be interviewed is not available on several attempted contacts, is recently deceased, or is not otherwise available, then attempts to gather information on this person should still be pursued through a close relative or other reputable source. This is important to be able to stick as closely to the random nature of the sample, and also to provide for the most representative data.

10. Confidentially will be stressed throughout the entire training and interview process. A release of information/statement of rights and expectations will be provided and signed by each person interviewed. The interviewers must assure the respondents that the facts will not be repeated to anyone outside of the interview context. This is imperative to ensure the most accurate survey information. Further, the questionnaires will not be linked with the respondent's name once the data have been collected.

The sample will be drawn from the tribal roles using enrollment number. The number will be matched with a name, the person will then be contacted, interviewed, and nothing except a questionnaire I.D. Number (different than the census number) will be on the questionnaire. The actual sample list of names and census numbers will not be connected with the questionnaires except on a master list which will be kept by the research agency, and all lists and questionnaires will be locked in a file cabinet at U.N.M. - C.A.S.A.A. Once the data have been fed into the computer for processing and have been backed up with extra data files, then the actual questionnaires will be destroyed. All of the results of the study will be reported in aggregate form, and therefore will be no risk to the individual.

11. The time frame of this study will be nine months as proposed here. This time frame will ensure that U.N.M. and the Navajo Nation can work together for the best quality data, usable results and a meaningful report.

Duties to be preformed by U.N.M. - C.A.S.A.A.

This proposal will commit U.N.M. - C.A.S.A.A. to performing the following tasks.

1. Prepare a draft of the interview schedule/questionnaire to be used in the study and work with the Behavioral Health Services personnel on the final content of the questionnaire.

2. Define the exact sampling procedures and select the sample.

3. Organize and provide instruction and training for the Navajo interviewers (who will be employed by the Tribe), on the interviewing techniques, sample gathering and other technical issues.

4. Perform the data entry, processing, and detailed analysis on University computers.

5. Write the final report and deliver it to the Department of Behavioral Health Services.

Other Considerations

This proposal assumes, based on the request for proposal originally issued by the Navajo Tribe, that the Navajo Tribe will: 1.) Employ the interviewers, 2.) Will pay for their transportation to the training session and lodging while there, 3.) And will pay for the interviewer's transportation and expenses necessary in locating and interviewing the respondents.

Personnel

The University of New Mexico will provide, with this proposal, the services of the principal investigator, Philip A. May, Ph.D. (resume attached), an administrative assistant, and at least two advanced level (master's degree plus further training) graduate students as program and research specialists (see budget). Further, it will be necessary to hire at least one and possibly two consultants who are very familiar with Navajo cultural issues as they affect this particular research project to assist in the training session.

All other participating personnel and their expenses will be borne by the Navajo Tribe.

A Final Consideration

It is the hope of U.N.M. - C.A.S.A.A. that the Navajo Nation, Department of Behavioral Health, can use this project to not only produce a meaningful and valid study, but also to raise the awareness of the population regarding:

1. The positive action which they can take by participating fully in this study,

2. The positive role they can play in the solution of the problem,

3. And, the promise of solving alcohol and substance abuse problems through comprehensive and specifically targeted public health measures based on this Navajo-specific prevalence study.

U.N.M. - C.A.S.A.A. proposes to lend its technical and professional support and guidance to this effort in order to further empower the Navajo Nation.

REFERENCES

Levy, Jerrold E. and Kunitz, Steven J. Indian Drinking. New York: Wiley Interscience, 1974.

May, Philip A. Substance Abuse and American Indians: Prevalence and Susceptibility. International Journal of the Addictions, 17, 1185-1209, 1982.

May, Philip A. Alcohol Abuse and Alcoholism Among American Indians: An Overview. In: Alcoholism in Minority Populations, Thomas D. Watts and Roosevelt Wright, Jr. (eds.). Springfield, Illinois: Charles C. Thomas, Publisher. 1989a.

May, Philip A. Assessment of Risk and Safety Variables for Adolescents in New Mexico: Comparative Ethnic Data. Manuscript prepared for the Health and Environment Division, State of New Mexico, Santa Fe, 1989b.

May, Philip A. and Smith, Matthew B. Some Navajo Indian Opinions About Alcohol Abuse and Prohibition: A Survey and Recommendations for Policy. Journal of Studies on Alcohol, 49: 324-334, 1988.

Oetting, Eugene R. and Beauvais, Fred. Epidemiology and Correlates of Alcohol Use among Indian Adolescents Living on Reservations. Paper presented at the NIAAA Conference on the Epidemiology of Alcohol Use and Abuse Among U.S. Ethnic Minorities, Bethesda, Maryland, September, 1985.

Winfree, L. Thomas and Griffiths, Curt T. Youth at Risk: Marijuana Use among Native American and Caucasion Youths. International Journal of the Addictions, 20(10), 1495-1508, 1983.

Budget

	Wage	Fringe*	Total	
Personnel:				
Philip A. May, Ph.D., Principal Investigator (20 days @ 290)	5800	1276	7076	
Phyllis Trujillo, B.A. Administrative Assistant (30 days @ 62)	1860	409	2270	
Graduate Student, Project Coordinator (70 days @ 88)	6160	123	6283	
Graduate Student, Data Specialist (70 days @ 88)	6160	123	6283	
				21,912.00
Consultants:				
2 consultants @ $250, 2 days each			1,000	
Consultant per diem, 2 days @75.00 and 2 days @ 25.00			200	
Consultant travel - 2 trips to Window Rock (325 mi. ea. @ .26)			169	
				1,369.00
Travel:				
5 trips to Window Rock (@325 mi. ea., @ .25)			406	
4 nights lodging @ 50.00			200	
10 days per diem @ 25.00			250	
				856.00
Data Processing:				
Computer use costs, printing of questionnaires, use of scanner, paper, materials, supplies, and miscellaneous.			2,000	
				2,000.00
Other:				
Telephone use			100	
Postage			50	
Office Supplies			50	
				200.00
		TOTAL DIRECT		26,337.00
		INDIRECT @ 48.5%**		12,773.00
		TOTAL COSTS		39,110.00

* Fringe Benefits at U.N.M. are 22% for faculty and Staff and 2% for graduate students.

** Indirect rate is the federally approved rate for U.N.M. research projects.

Biographical Sketch

Philip A. May, Ph.D.
SS# 217-48-4442
Professor of Sociology and Psychiatry
University of New Mexico
Albuquerque, NM 87131
(505) 768-0100

Degrees:

A.B.	1969	Catawba College, Salisbury, NC	Sociology
M.A.	1971	Wake Forest University, Winston-Salem, NC	Sociology
Ph.D.	1976	University of Montana, Missoula, MT	Sociology

Honors:

1966-69	Sigma Pi Alpha (Honorary Language Fraternity)
1969	Who's Who Among Students in American Colleges and Universities
1969-70	Wake Forest University Fellowship
1982	Chair, Enforcement Committee, N.M. Governor's Task Force on Alcohol A and Driving
1982	Certificate of Appreciation, National Indian Health Board
1982	American Men and Women of Science
1985	Certificate of Appreciation, N.M. Indian Nurse Association
1988	Who's Who in Sociology
1986 and 1988	Faculty Member of the Year, UNM Sociology Graduate Student Associa Award (1st and 3rd Annual Recipient)

Experience:

1969-Summer	Research Appointment, U.S.P.H.S. (COSTEP), NIMH Center for Studie: Suicide Prevention.
1970-1973	Staff Sociologist, U.S.P.H.S. (Commissioned Corps), Community Me Health Program, P.H.S. Indian Hospital, Pine Ridge, SD.
1970-1973	Instructor of Sociology (part-time), Oglala Sioux Tribal Commu College, Pine Ridge, SD.
1973-1976	NIMH Criminology Traineeship, University of Montana, Missoula, MT 59
1976-1978	Director of Health Statistics and Research and Director of Window Office, Navajo Health Authority, Window Rock, AZ 86515.
1978-1982	Assistant Professor of Sociology, University of New Mexico.
1979-1985	Program Director, National Indian Fetal Alcohol Syndrome Preven Program and I.H.S. Pilot Project on F.A.S.
1980-1986	Program Director, NIMH Ph.D. Training Program in Research on Dev Behavior, University of New Mexico.
1982-1989	Associate Professor of Sociology, University of New Mexico
1987 (Jan-Aug)	Head, Department of Sociology, Anthropology, and Criminal Justice, Mon State University, Bozeman, MT 57717.
1989-Present	Director, New Mexico Access to Research Careers (NMARC Program).
1989-Present	Professor of Sociology
1990-Present	Director, Center on Alcoholism, Substance Abuse and Addictions (CAS University of New Mexico, and Professor of Psychiatry.

Contracts and Grants Awarded: (Selected)

"Analysis of Existing Alcohol Programs for the Navajo Area and Suggestions for Future Programs." USPHS, Division of Indian Health, Window Rock, AZ, 1978-1979, $49,944, # 78-0121.

"Auto Accident Analysis and Implementation for the Navajo Nation." USPHS, Division of In Health, Window Rock, AZ, 1978-1979, $35,129, #63A0000010, C2.

"Ph.D. Training Program in Research on Crime and Delinquency." Continuation gra: N.I.M.H., Center for Studies on Crime and Deliquency, Rockville, MD, 1981-1 $82,303, #5-T01-MH15219-05.

78-786 - 94 -- 7

"Fetal Alcohol Syndrome Demonstration Project." U.S.P.H.S. Division of Indian Health, Rockville, MD, 1980-1981, $126,312, #HRA 240-81-0002.
"National Indian Fetal Alcohol Syndrome Prevention Program." U.S.P.H.S. Division of Indian Health, Rockville, MD, 1983-1985, $308,447, #HRSA 240-83-0064.
"Ph.D Training in Applied Research on Deviant Behavior." N.I.M.H., Center for Studies of Crime and Delinquency, Rockville, MD, 1983-1986, $165,921, #1-T32-MH1744.
"Research Career Program for New Mexico Minorities." ADAMHA-MARC Program in Alcohol, Drug Abuse, and Mental Health Research, 1989-1994, $715,722, SRCM(M), #T34-MH19101.

Journal Articles and Book Chapters:

Adolescent Suicide at an Indian Reservation. American Journal of Orthopsychiatry, 44:43-49, 1974. with Larry Dizmang, Jane Watson, John Bopp.
Suicide and the American Indian. Psychiatric Annals, 4:22-28,1974. with Larry H. Dizmang.
Arrests, Alcohol and Alcohol Legalization among an American Indian Tribe. Plains Anthropologist, 20:129-134, 1975.
Explanations of Native American Drinking: A Literature Review, Plains Anthropologist, A22:223-232, 1977.
A Survey of Tribal Alcohol Statutes, American Indian Law Review, (51):217-228, 1977.
A Navajo Health Consumer Survey, Medical Care, 18(12):1183-1195, 1980. with Thomas Stewart and Anita Muneta.
Recruitment and Retention of Federal Physicians on the Navajo Reservation, The Social Science Journal, 19(4):47-66, 1982. with Rodney L. Brod and Thomas J. Stewart.
Contemporary Crime and the American Indian: A Survey and Analysis of the Literature. Plains Anthropologist 27(97):225238,1982.
Substance Abuse and American Indians: Prevalence and Susceptibility. International Journal of the Addictions, 17(7):1185-1209, 1982.
A Pilot Project on Fetal Alcohol Syndrome for American Indians. Alcohol Health and Research World, 7:3-9, 1983. with Karen J. Hymbaugh.
Demographic and Epidemiologic Transition among the Navajo Indians. Social Biology, 30:(1):1-16, 1983. with David w. Broudy.
Fetal Alcohol Syndrome among American Indians of the Southwest. Social Biology, 30(4):374-487, 1983. with K.h. Hymbaugh, J.M. Aase, and J.M. Samet.
Inhalant Abuse and Juvenile Delinquency: A Control Study in Albuquerque, New Mexico. International Journal of the Addictions, 19(8):789-803, 1984. with Barbara j. F. Reed.
Native American Suicide in New Mexico, 1957-79: A Comparative Study. Human Organization, 45(4):296-301, 1986. with Nancy W. Van Winkle.
Alcohol and Drug Abuse Prevention Programs for American Indians: Needs and Opportunities. Journal of Studies on Alcohol, 47(3):187-195, 1986.
Suicide and Self-Destruction among American Indian Youths, American Indian and Alaska Native Mental Health, 11:52-69, 1987.
The Health Status of Indian Children: Problems and Prevention in Early Life. pp. 244-283, In: Manson, S. and Dinges, N. (eds.). Health and Behavior: A Research Agenda for American Indians and Alaska Natives. Denver, Colorado, Health Sciences University Press, 1988.
Navajo Indian Opinions about Alcohol Abuse and Prohibition: A Survey, Journal of Studies on Alcohol, 49(4):324-344, 1988. with Matthew B. Smith.
Mental Health and Alcohol Abuse Indicators in the Albuquerque Area of Indian Health Service: A Chart Review, Journal of American Indian and Alaska Native Mental Health Research, 2(1):33-46, 1988.
Alcohol Abuse and Alcoholism among American Indians: An Overiew. pp 95-119, In: Alcoholism in Minority Populations, Thomas D. Watts and Roosevelt Wright, Jr. (eds.). Springfield, IL, Charles C. Thomas Publishers, 1989.
Profile of Abused and Neglected Indian Children in the Southwest, Child Abuse and Neglect: The International Journal, 13:449-461, 1989. with Carol C. Lujan, Leymra DeBruyn, and Michael E. Bird.
Motor Vehicle Crashes and Alcohol among American Indian and Alaska Natives, pp 207-223. In: Office of the Surgeon General, U.S. Public Health Service, The Surgeon General's Workshop in Drunk Driving: Background Papers. Washington, D.C., U.S. Department of Health and Human Services, 1989.
A Macro-Level Fetal Alcohol Syndrome Prevention Program for American Indians and Alaska Natives: Description and Evaluation, Journal of Studies on Alcohol, 50(6):508-518, 1989. with Karen J. Hymbaugh.
Suicide and Suicide Attempts among American Indians and Alaska Natives: A Bibliography, Omega, 2(3):199-214, 1990.

Alcohol Policy Considerations for Indian Reservations and Bordertown Communities, <u>Journa</u> <u>American Indian and Alaska Native Mental Health Research</u>, in press.
Indian Adolescent Suicide: The Epidemiologic Picture in New Mexico, with Nancy Westlake Winkle, <u>American Indian and Alaska Native Mental Health Research</u>, in press.
An Update on American Indian Suicide in New Mexico, 1980-1987, with Nancy Westlake Winkle, submitted for review.

<u>Applied Monographs</u> (selected):

<u>Navajo Comparative Health Services Evaluation Project</u>. Navajo Health Authority, 1977, pp. with D. W. Broudy, M. Austin, K. Battese and M. Hudson.
<u>Motor Vehicle Accidents on the Navajo Reservation: 1973-75</u>. Navajo Health Authority, 1 104 pp. with Phillip S. Katz.
<u>Suicide and Suicide Attempts among American Indians and Alaska Natives: An Annot Bibliography.</u> U.S.P.H.S., Indian Health Service, 1987, 147 pp. second edition, 1 201 pp.

Phyllis Trujillo	Staff Assistant	March 7, 1961

The University of New Mexico, Albuq., NM	A.A.	1981	Secretarial Studies/ Office Supervision
The University of New Mexico, Albuq., NM	B.S.	1984	Business Education

title	employer
Receptionist/Secretary June 1985 - May 1986	The Rehabilitation Center 1023 Stanford Dr. NE Albuquerque, NM 87106
Bookkeeper May 1986 - October 1987	The Rehabilitation Center 1023 Stanford Dr. NE Albuquerque, NM 87106
Office Manager October 1987 - February 1990	The Rehabilitation Center RCI Enterprises 2901 Edith NE Albuquerque, NM 87107
Clerical Specialist V February 1990 - July 1990	The Center on Alcoholism, Substance Abuse and Addictions 2350 alamo SE Albuquerque, NM 87106
Staff Assistant/Admin. August 1990 - present	The Center on Alcoholism, Substance Abuse and Addictions 2350 alamo SE Albuquerque, NM 87106

VITA
(January 1993)

Ann M. Del Vecchio, M.A., N.C.C.
1333 Columbia N.E.
Albuquerque, New Mexico 87106
(505) 255-2199

<u>Education</u>

Current: course-work for Doctorate in Research Methodology through the Department of Educational Foundations at the University of New Mexico is in progress. Major study concentration is in quantitative methodology. Minor course of study is in Cognitive Psychology.

M.A. Counseling, May 1988, University of New Mexico Outstanding Academic Achievement Award for the Class of 1988, Master's thesis: **"World View and Political Activism in a Southwestern Multicultural Sample"**.

B.S. Psychology, May 1976, University of New Mexico Magna Cum Laude, Honor's thesis: **"Reactions to Artistic and Experimental Stimuli"**.

<u>Practicum Internship</u>

Cognitive assessment at the Bernalillo County Detention Center, January 1988 to May 1988. Primary duties included preliminary screening of residents identified by the Education Director using the Bender Visual Motor Gestalt Test and the Wechsler Adult Intelligence Test- Revised for learning disabilities, organic impairment, or other cognitive difficulties. If indicated by preliminary testing, further testing was done. Some individual therapy, and stress management,with residents who had been tested was done during this internship as well.

<u>Employment</u>

July 1992 to current: Research Assistant, Center on Alcoholism, Substance Abuse and Addictions (CASAA), Voices of Indian Teens Project

Responsibilities: Collect and analyze data from rural, Native American high school students related to risk factors for alcohol and substance abuse. Report results of bi-annual data collection to school sites.

June 1992 to current: Research Assistant, Center on Alcoholism, Substance Abuse and Addictions (CASAA),

Employment

Taos Pueblo Community Partnership Evaluation

Responsibilities: Manage and analyze process and outcome evaluation data. Prepare evaluation reports including graphic data representation. Provide technical assistance to the partnership as needed.

September 1990 to May 1992: Graduate Assistant, Research Advisory Services.

Responsibilities: Teach small group review sessions which cover introductory statistics and IBM-7171 mainframe access and use, tutoring students in statistics and research design, completing special projects analyses, grant writing, program planning and evaluation, technical assistance to College of Education students, faculty, and staff with research questions.

September 1990 to June 30, 1991: Project Coordinator, A.W.A.R.E.- N.M.

Responsibilities: Planning and implementation of Project objectives, including regional activities organizational newsletter, two conferences per year, and membership. Develop and maintain positive relationship with Advisory Board, Project Director, the SDE Project Monitor, school districts, and project participants. Manage Project budget, prepare and submit proposals and quarterly reports. Design and maintain database of information to enhance and to implement the project goals and activities. Wrote and submitted the proposal for 1991-1992 funding to the State Department of Education; project was funded for $32,000.

May 1988 to June 30, 1990: Counselor, and Evaluation Specialist, Genesis Women's Center.

Responsibilities: Provide individual and group therapy to adult, female felony offenders and their families. Managed a caseload of twelve which involved treatment planning, job development, intensive supervision, and case management. Analysis of successful versus unsuccessful graduates indicated that 60% of my caseload graduated the program successfully. The program overall, had a 50% success rate. Provided all cognitive and personality assessment for the entire program's caseload. Supervised interns from

<u>Employment</u>

a variety of training backgrounds in individual, family, and group counseling. Evaluated intern performance for internship coordinators. Provided in-service training to co-workers and Department of Corrections staff. Calculated program's statistics for Department of Corrections accountability and prepared quarterly reports detailing caseload progress. Limited grant and proposal preparation (United Way, N.I.D.A.).

June 1982 to June 1988, Child Care Worker, Children's Psychiatric Hospital.

Responsibilities: Provision of direct care to 14 year old emotionally disturbed adolescents in a hospital, milieu setting. Implemented treatment plans, directed group activities, and group milieu therapy, managed weekend activities money, taught social, life, and communication skills as part of a treatment team.

September 1981 to September 1987, Newsletter Editor, and Board Member, Parentcraft, Family and Children's Services.

Responsibilities: Organized parenting information, recruited writers for each issue, researched and wrote articles, proof read and approved final copy, updated mailing list. As a Board Member, responsibilities included the hiring, supervision,and direction of the agency director. Reviewed and approved the monthly budget. Provided fiscal, personnel, and programmatic policy, and procedure to the agency. Provided short and long range planning, fund-raising, and merger negotiations. During tenure as Parentcraft's President of the Board of Directors, merger negotiations with Family and Children's Services were completed. Served as a member of the Board for the combined agencies following the merger.

<u>Contract Experience</u>

October 1992 to current: Research Associate, Evaluation Assistance Center-West

June 1992 to November 1992: Research Consultant, Bernalillo County Maternal/Child Health Needs Assessment

January 1992 to December 1992: Research Consultant, Indian Health Service

January 1992 to December 1992: Statistics Consultant, Learning Resources International

October 1991 to December 1991: Project Evaluation Coordinator, Bilingual Special Education, Federally funded project in the Albuquerque Public Schools.

September 1990 to November 1991: Research Consultant, "Fighting Back Initiative" (Funded through the Robert Wood Johnson Foundation).

January 1991 to May 1991: Research Consultant, Titan Corporation; 21st Century Project Evaluation

January 1991, Research Consultant, BETA Group

January 1990, Member of the Habilitation Review Team for Protection and Advocacy

<u>Testing Experience</u>

WAIS-R	Rorschach
WISC-R	MMPI
WRAT-R	16-PF
SOI	CPI
Woodcock-Johnson	Millon (MCMI)

Thematic Apperception Test
Vineland Adaptive Behavior Scale
Bender Visual Motor Gestalt Test
Revised Beta Examination II
Strong Campbell Interest Inventory
Myers Briggs Type Indicator
Behavioral assessment tools for anxiety, anger depression, acculturation, drug and alcohol abuse, suicide attention deficit disorder, etc.

<u>Presentations</u>

Evaluation Assistance Center-West: Oklahoma Association for Bilingual Education, November, 1992
"Teaching Test Taking Skills to Limited English Proficient Students"
"Title VII Evaluation Guidelines for Bilingual Education Project Directors"

Research Advisory Services Review Sessions on the following topics:

- Research design
- Basic Algebra
- Samples & Populations; Distributions
- Independent *t* -tests and *z*-scores
- Dependent *t*-tests
- Association measures; Correlation, Chi Square
- Analysis of Variance (ANOVA)

MUSIC; Terminal Language for the Mainframe

New Mexico Corrections Department Workshops:
Active Listening: Asking open ended questions"
Genesis Women's Center, February 1989
"CoDependency and Women Offenders"
Department of Corrections, District II Office
June 25, 1990
"Reading a Psychological Evaluation"
Department of Corrections, District II Office
June 26, 1990
Volunteer Training and Orientation
Community Involved Parole/Probation Program
Wednesdays, June 1990

Training

"The Crisis of Children Exposed to Drugs and Alcohol" University of New Mexico, School of Medicine, C.A.S.A.A., Department of Psychiatry, Office of Continuing Medical Education, August 13-15, 1992

"Southwestern Psychiatric Symposium on Substance Abuse"
UNM School of Medicine, C.A.S.A.A., Department of Psychiatry, Office of Continuing Medical Education
February 1991

"Psychotherapeutic Interventions with Spanish and Native American Children"
University of New Mexico Continuing Medical Education:
May 1987
May 1988
May 1989
June 1990

"Substance Abuse and Corrections"
Shaening and Associates
October 1989

Certification National Board Counselor Certification: # 21462

Affiliations

American Psychological Association
National Council on Measurement in Education
American Educational Research Association

References References are available upon request.

Interview Protocol

DRAFT

Please introduce yourself using the traditional Navajo form, including identification of your parents' clans. After you have completed your introduction and the respondent has replied, explain your purpose.

"I am working on a survey sponsored by the Navajo Tribe's Department of Behavioral Health Services. You should have received a letter from Behavioral Health Services telling you about this survey. (have a copy of the letter for the respondent available) The answers to the questions we ask will be kept strictly confidential and no names are connected with this survey. Most of the questions are about alcohol, tobacco, and other drugs. The results of this study will be the main source of information for the Navajo Tribe on alcohol and drug experience, attitudes, and knowledge. This information will be used for important prevention and intervention services for the Navajo Tribe.

Please use the paragraph above as a guideline for your explanation.

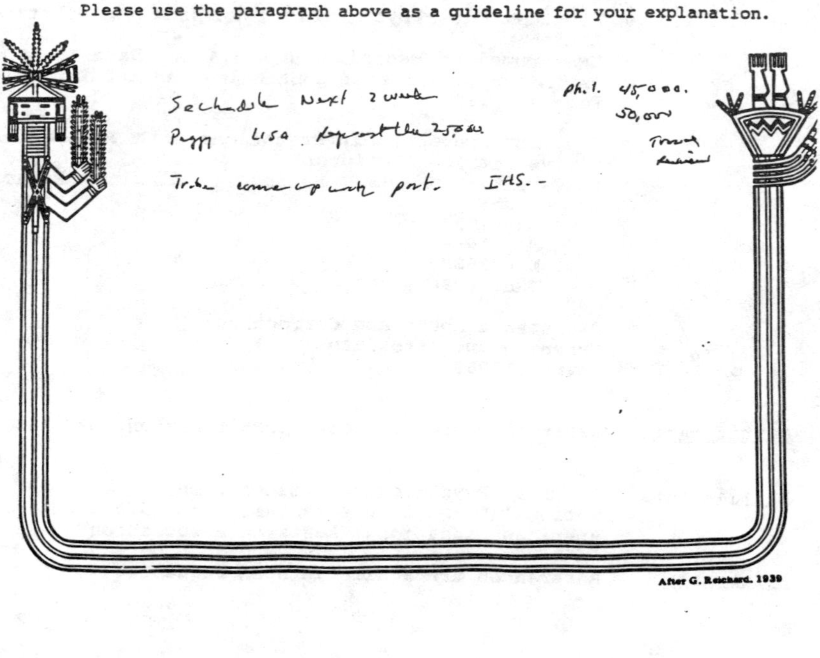

Schedule Next 2 weeks

Peggy Lisa. [illegible] 25,000

Tribe come up with part. IHS.-

Ph. 1. 45,000.
50,000

After G. Reichard, 1939

Interview Protocol

Please introduce yourself using the traditional Navajo form, including identification of your parents' clans. After you have completed your introduction and the respondent has replied, explain your purpose.

"I am working on a survey sponsored by the Navajo Tribe's Department of Behavioral Health Services. You should have received a letter from Behavioral Health Services telling you about this survey. (have a copy of the letter for the respondent available) The answers to the questions we ask will be kept strictly confidential and no names are connected with this survey. Most of the questions are about alcohol, tobacco, and other drugs. The results of this study will be the main source of information for the Navajo Tribe on alcohol and drug experience, attitudes, and knowledge. This information will be used for important prevention and intervention services for the Navajo Tribe.

Please use the paragraph above as a guideline for your explanation.

If the respondent is Native American but not Navajo, please ask them to identify their tribe/s. If the respondent belongs to another ethnic group please print the name of this ethnic group

The interviewer will mark the respondent's sex on the first line of the interview book.

Next ask the respondent to tell you his/her birth date and print this clearly on the line. Next ask the respondent for his/her age in years.

The first section is called "site of interview". Although we anticipate that most of the people to be interviewed will be on the Navajo Reservation, we have divided this question into three separate sections. Please print the name of the reservation on the line by "reservation". Then ask the respondent to tell you the name of his or her Chapter House of residence. Next ask the respondent to tell you the name of their Chapter House of enrollment. The next line is for you to fill out if the interview is with someone who resides in Gallup, Tuba City, or any other community, town, or city, not in the Reservation. Please PRINT all this information clearly.

There are two lines available for occupation. Please use the first line to record wage work occupations. Examples of wage work are seamstress, cook, teacher, truck driver, sales person, scientist, lawyer, and carpenter. The second line which says "other occupations" is for work which is Navajo traditional. Examples of this are herbalist, weaver, potter, beader, medicine man. Some things will fit in both categories, like sheepherder and farmer. Please write these occupations on both lines.

The next block is for education. Please mark the highest level of education completed by the respondent. Technical certification is for a trade such as welding. Please be sure to find out if the respondent has completed high school or has a GED so that you may mark the correct category for those respondents who have technical certification in a trade.

Ask the respondent to estimate his/her annual income and check the category for this.

The next questions ask the respondent to identify the language they speak at home, at work, and with friends. If they ask you to clarify, please tell them most of the time. If they use more than one language regularly in these situations, please mark all the languages they use.

If the respondent has lived off the reservation for more than one year, please write out the number of years.

The next questions are about religion and spiritual beliefs. If the respondent states that he/she practices traditional ceremonies and prayers, please ask them which ones and write this information on the lines provided. The next question is about other spiritual beliefs. Please mark the appropriate category.

Question 21 asks the respondent to answer whether or not he/she would name a child (if or when they become a parent) with a traditional name. Question 22 asks the respondent to identify the type of health care provider he/she prefers. If they offer an answer not covered by these choices, please write their answer down in the margin. All the completed surveys will be read carefully. If you have additional information to include write it in the margins or on the back of the page.

Question 23 asks the respondent about marital status. Check the appropriate choice. Finally, question 24 asks for the total number of people living in the household and question 25 asks for the total number of dependents. Fill this information in on the lines provided.

Sex: Female _____
Male _____

Interviewer will note dwelling type: 1.Hogan
2.Pueblo
3.Other traditional home?

1) Mark type of housing:
_____ one or two story frame
_____ mud covered hogan
_____ log hogan
_____ lumber hogan
_____ combination hogan and frame
_____ trailer
_____ H.U.D. housing
_____ other type of home

2) What is your mother's clan? ____________________

3) What is your father's clan? ____________________

4) Tribe, if the respondent is not Navajo: ____________________

5) Ethnic group if the respondent is not Native American:

____

What is your birth-date? ____________________

6) Age: __________ years

Site of Interview:

7) Reservation: ____________________

8) Community (Chapter House of Residence) ____________________

9) Community (Chapter House Enrollment) ____________________

10) Places: ____________________

11) What is your occupation/s: ____________________

12) Other occupations: ____________________

page 2

Education categories: (coded in grade block)

- ___ Kindergarten through 3'rd grade
- ___ 4'th through 6'th grade
- ___ 7'th through 9'th
- ___ 9'th through 12'th
- ___ Technical Cert. w/o high school diploma
- ___ High school diploma
- ___ GED
- ___ Technical Cert. with high school diploma
- ___ Associate degree
- ___ BS/BA
- ___ MS/MA
- ___ MD/Law
- ___ Ph.D./Ed.D.

13) Annual Family Income:

- under $10,000/yr. _____
- $10,001-19,000 _____
- $19,001-34,000 _____
- $34,001-50,000 _____
- above $50,001/yr. _____

14) Language you speak at home:

- English _____
- Spanish _____
- Navajo _____
- Zuni _____
- Hopi _____
- Other __________

15) Language you speak at work:

- English _____
- Spanish _____
- Navajo _____
- Zuni _____
- Hopi _____
- Other __________

16) Language you speak with friends:

- English _____
- Spanish _____
- Navajo _____
- Zuni _____
- Hopi _____
- Other __________

17) Have you ever lived off the reservation for more than one year?

yes _____ no _____

18) If the answer is yes, how long? __________________________ years

page 3

19) Do you practice your tribe's traditional prayers/ceremonies?

yes _____ no ______

Which of your tribe's traditional prayers/ceremonies do you practice?

____

____

____

20) How often do you practice your tribe's traditional prayers/ceremonies?

_____ daily _____ monthly
_____ weekly _____ yearly or less often

21) What is your spiritual affiliation?

_____ traditional Navajo _____ Catholic
_____ Native American Church _____ Protestant
_____ Later Day Saints _____ Assembly of God
___________________________________ Other

22) When you become a parent will you give the baby or have the baby given a traditional name? _____ yes _____ no

23) Please identify the type or types of health care providers you would prefer if ill or in need of counsel.

_____ a traditional healer (medicine man/woman)
_____ a medical doctor
_____ both

24) Marital Status: Single _____
Married _____
Living with someone _____
Separated _____
Divorced _____
Widowed _____

25) Total number in household ___________________________________

26) Total number of dependents in household _____________________

page 4

27) Does anyone in your immediate family have a problem with alcohol? _____ yes _____ no

28) If you marked yes, what relation are they? ________________

29) Do any of your friends have a problem with alcohol?

_____ yes _____ no

30) If you yes, how many? ______________________

****
The following questions are being asked of everyone. Please help us/me by answering based on your experience.
****

31) How old were you the first time you had a glass of beer or wine or drink of liquor, such as whiskey, gin, or scotch? (do not include childhood sips you might have had from an older person's drink).

______________________________ years

32) How old were you when you first began to drink beer wine or liquor once a month or more often?

______________________________ years

The following questions all apply to the last 30 days.

33) On how many different days did you have one or more drinks of beer, wine, or liquor?

____

34) How many drinks did you usually have in a day on the days that you drank during the past 30 days?

______________________________ drinks

35) On how many days did you have five or more drinks of beer, wine. or liquor, on the same occasion during the past 30 days?

______________________________ days

page 5

36) What is the most you had to drink on any one day you drank beer, wine, or liquor during the past 30 days?

____

37) How many days did you have this number of drinks of beer, wine, or liquor in the past 30 days?

________________________________ days

In the past 12 months

38) On the average how often in the past 12 months have you had any alcoholic beverage, that is, beer, wine, or liquor?

_____ yes _____ no

39) How many times during the past 12 months have you gotten high or drunk on alcohol (beer, wine, liquor)?

________________________________ times

40) On those occasions when you drink alcohol is it usually

_____ beer
_____ wine
_____ liquor
_____ hairspray
_____ mouthwash
_____ rubbing alcohol
_____ other

41) How many drinks of beer, wine, or liquor does it take to get an average person drunk?

____

How can you tell if a person is drunk?

____

____

____

____

page 6	yes	no
42) I get upset and attack when drinking.	X	X
43) I get into a heated argument while drinking.	X	X
44) I have stayed away from work or school because of a hangover.	X	X
45) I was high or a little drunk on the job or at school.	X	X
46) I lost a job or nearly lost one because of drinking.	X	X
47) My wife/husband or girl/boy friend told me I should cut down on my drinking.	X	X
48) A relative other than my husband/wife told me I should cut down on my drinking.	X	X
49) Friends told me I should cut down on my drinking.	X	X
50) I tossed down several drinks to get a quicker effect.	X	X
51) I may be an alcoholic or become one.	X	X
52) I stayed drunk for more than one day at a time.	X	X
53) Once I start drinking it is difficult for me to stop.	X	X
54) I have awakened unable to remember some of the things I had done while drinking the day before.	X	X
55) I had a quick drink or so when no one was looking.	X	X
56) I often took a drink first thing in the morning.	X	X
57) My hands shook a lot after drinking the day before.	X	X
58) Sometimes I got high or a little drunk when drinking by myself.	X	X
59) I kept on drinking after promising to quit.	X	X
60) I have been injured while drinking.	X	X

page 7

	yes	no
61) I have physically hurt others while drinking?	X	X
62) I have friends who have been injured as a result of someone else's drinking.	X	X

(special code section)

If the respondent does not drink, and never did drink, please mark the questionnaire here. ______________________________

	cigarettes	alcohol	inhalants	marijuana	cocaine/crack	prescription drugs	heroin	PCP/angel dust	other
Please mark which of the following drugs you use:	X	X	X	X	X	X	X	X	X
During the past twelve months for which drugs have you been unable to cut down on your use please mark all that apply:	X	X	X	X	X	X	X	X	X
During the past twelve months for which drugs have you needed larger amounts to get the same effect:	X	X	X	X	X	X	X	X	X
During the past twelve months which drugs have you used every day or almost daily for two weeks or more in a row? - mark all that apply:	X	X	X	X	X	X	X	X	X
Which drugs have you felt that you needed or were dependent on in the past twelve months - mark all that apply	X	X	X	X	X	X	X	X	X
) For which drugs have you had withdrawal symptoms: that is, felt sick because you stopped or cut down your use during the past twelve months :	X	X	X	X	X	X	X	X	X

page 9

69) Have you ever used a needle to get any drug injected under your skin, into a muscle, or into a vein for non medical reasons?

_____ yes _____ no

70) When was the most recent time you used a needle to inject drugs for any non medical reasons?

____

71) If you use inhalants, please identify which ones:

gasoline/lighter fluid _____
spray paints _____
metallic spray paints _____
rubber cement _____
markers _____
lacquer thinner/paint solvents _____
correction fluids _____
hair spray/other aerosol sprays _____
other _____

72) When do you use inhalants? _______________________________________

73) In your opinion, are drugs a problem in your community?

_____ yes _____ no

74) If drugs are a problem please mark which ones (mark all that apply)?

cigarettes _____
alcohol _____
inhalants _____
marijuana _____
cocaine/crack _____
prescription drugs _____
heroin _____
PCP/angel dust _____
other _____

75) Should alcohol be legalized on your reservation?

_____ yes _____ no

76) In your opinion, is alcohol a problem in your community?

_____ yes _____ no

page 10

Do you believe that drinking <u>three</u> or more drinks a day puts a person at risk for:

	agree strongly		undecided		disagree strongly
77) accidental injury	1	2	3	4	5
78) problems at work	1	2	3	4	5
79) birth defects	1	2	3	4	5
80) getting into legal trouble	1	2	3	4	5
81) relationship problems	1	2	3	4	5
82) blackouts	1	2	3	4	5
83) cirrhosis	1	2	3	4	5
84) DT's	1	2	3	4	5
85) brain damage	1	2	3	4	5
86) death	1	2	3	4	5
87) seizures	1	2	3	4	5
88) heart disease	1	2	3	4	5

Several alcohol related issues are listed below. Please mark whether or not you feel these issues are a problem in your community.

	agree strongly		undecided		disagree strongly
89) sale of alcohol to minors	1	2	3	4	5
90) sale of alcohol at gas stations	1	2	3	4	5
91) happy hours at bars & restaurants	1	2	3	4	5
92) advertising of alcoholic beverages	1	2	3	4	5
93) family violence due to alcohol	1	2	3	4	5
94) child abuse/neglect due to alcohol	1	2	3	4	5
95) crime due to alcohol	1	2	3	4	5
96) problems or injuries at work	1	2	3	4	5
97) drinking & driving	1	2	3	4	5
98) individual drinking problems	1	2	3	4	5
99) number of alcohol outlets	1	2	3	4	5
100) public intoxication	1	2	3	4	5
101) protective custody	1	2	3	4	5
102) bootlegging sales	1	2	3	4	5
103) inefficient police enforcement of laws against bootlegging	1	2	3	4	5
104) penalties too low for bootlegging	1	2	3	4	5

page 11

105) Have you had a problem with alcohol in the past? _____ yes
_____ no

106) If you are now abstinent, have you been abstinent for more than a year? _____ yes
_____ no

107) How did you quit?
_____ in-patient treatment
_____ out-patient treatment
_____ both
_____ neither
_____ with the help of a healer
_____ cold turkey
_____ with the help of family and friends

Why did you quit?____

____

____

____

Why do you think some people drink so much alcohol that they become very sick?

____

____

____

____

National Center for Substance Abuse Treatment - IHS

Navajo Project Deadlines

Publication	March 15	} 3 weeks
Technical Assistance	3 weeks ending April 7	
Receipt of Application	June 15	} 3 months (Publication to Receipt of Application)
Review	July	
Site Visit	August	
De brief NCSAT	August 25	
Award	September 15	} 6 months (Publication to Award)

INTRA-AGENCY AGREEMENT
DEPARTMENT OF HEALTH AND HUMAN SERVICES
PUBLIC HEALTH SERVICE
INDIAN HEALTH SERVICE AND
CENTER FOR SUBSTANCE ABUSE TREATMENT/
SUBSTANCE ABUSE AND MENTAL HEALTH SERVICES ADMINISTRATION

I. PURPOSE

The purpose of this agreement is to facilitate collaborative activities between the U.S. Public Health Service, Indian Health Services (IHS) and the U.S. Public Health Service, Center for Substance Abuse Treatment (CSAT).

II. SCOPE

CSAT and IHS will work together to expand access to effective addiction treatment services for American Indians and Alaskan Natives (AI/AN) based on the following understanding:

A. CSAT and IHS will endeavor to improve working relationships between the Tribal Authorities and Single State Agencies for Alcohol and Drug Abuse in each State; specific objectives include:

- Increasing the number of treatment programs serving AI/AN that are eligible for licensure by appropriate State licensure agencies.

- Ensuring that the needs of Native Americans are addressed through State activities sponsored under the CSAT State Systems Development Program (SSDP); specifically, ensuring that State incidence and prevalence assessments capture the treatment for Native Americans factors appropriately in the development of State Strategic plans.

B. CSAT and IHS will work together to improve the overall quality of programs for the treatment of Native Americans by accomplishing the following:

- Involving counselors who work in IHS-sponsored or Tribal-sponsored treatment programs in CSAT's National Substance Abuse Counselor Training Program.

- Including IHS representatives on Federal Resource Panels which oversee the development of CSAT's Treatment Improvement Protocol Statement (TIPS).

- Sharing the latest technology for the treatment of addiction and addiction-related illnesses.

- Jointly developing guidelines and training material fo: practitioners involved in the treatment of Native Americans, and disseminating these materials to the field.

- Ensuring that programs which focus on the treatment needs of Native Americans are clearly eligible to appl; for CSAT demonstration grants.

- Increasing the number of Native American treatment agencies that apply to CSAT for demonstration grants by: 1) jointly providing generic pre-application technical assistance to potential applicants; and 2) jointly educating IHS staff and IHS-sponsored treatment programs regarding the CSAT mission and CSAT programs structure.

- Ensuring that practitioners who are expert in the treatment of Native Americans participate in the revie of applications received by CSAT and ensuring that CSA expert reviewers participate in the review of application received by IHS.

- Ensuring that CSAT and IHS staff are cross-trained in subjects associated with: 1) clinical efficacy; 2) cultural/ethnic sensitivity; and 3) administration, monitoring and licensing practices.

C. CSAT and IHS will work to ensure that a portion of new CSAT demonstration program funds will be used in conjunction wit IHS resources to support projects that expand and/or enhanc treatment alternatives for Native Americans, as follows:

For FY 1993

- CSAT will endeavor to support a minimum of six Native American treatment projects under the auspices of its Critical Populations and Criminal Justice programs; a special effort will be made to support projects that address the needs of Native American women, adolescent and young adults and victims of alcohol and drug related birth defects.

- CSAT will work with the IHS to ensure that one major demonstration project, administered via cooperative agreement, is established in a small to moderately sized metropolitan setting where Native Americans constitute a large proportion of the target populatior

For FY 1994 and Beyond

Programs that focus on the treatment needs of Native Americans will be devised and implemented as appropriate given the volume of funds available and existing statutory and regulatory constraints, with the number and type of awards to be determined by mutual consent of the Directors, CSAT and IHS.

In order to facilitate the terms of this agreement, CSAT and IHS will establish a joint coordinating council to be composed of three representatives from each agency; the committee will meet on at least a quarterly basis and be charged with: 1) defining the demand for treatment among Native Americans from an epidemiological and etiological perspective; 2) devising specific plans for programs and technical assistance initiatives; and 3) making recommendations to the Directors, CSAT and IHS, for their review and approval.

III. DURATION OF AGREEMENT

This agreement will become effective immediately upon signatures of both parties and shall remain in effect through Fiscal Year 1995.

IV. MODIFICATION/CANCELLATION

This agreement may be modified at any time by mutual agreement in writing of both parties. Either party may terminate this agreement with 60 days written notice of the other party.

V. TRAVEL

Travel performed for the purpose of completing activities under this agreement is subject to allowances authorized in accordance with the Federal Travel regulations.

VI. DISSEMINATION OF INFORMATION

Information and data generated under this agreement will be published or disseminated based on the approval processes of both the IHS and the CSAT.

VII. AUTHORITY

This agreement is made under authority of the Economy Act, approved June 30, 1932 (31 USC 1535 and 1536).

VIII. **PROJECT OFFICERS**

The Indian Health Service and the Office for Treatment Improvement will appoint project officers for this agreement who will serve as the points of contact for the two organizations.

BY

INDIAN HEALTH SERVICE	OFFICE FOR TREATMENT IMPROVEMENT
SIGNATURE	SIGNATURE
DIRECTOR OF HEADQUARTERS OPERATIONS, IHS	Associate Administrator for Treatment Improvement, ADAMHA
TITLE	TITLE
23 Oct 1992	SEP 4 1992
DATE	DATE

NAVAJO NATION
DIVISION OF HEALTH

Testimony
on

Navajo Nation Health Issues:
Shiprock Field Hearing
April 8, 1994

INTRODUCTION

The Navajo Nation Division of Health which has the responsibility of developing and implementing comprehensive health care for the populace on the Navajo Nation is faced with copious number of health issues, but we are only sharing a few of our highly critical concerns and issues today for your consideration and support.

NAVAJO NATION TESTIMONY ON THE OUTBREAK OF HANTAVIRUS

Since May, and during part of the summer 1993 the Navajo Nation has experienced an outbreak of illness associated with Hantavirus infection evidenced by fever, headaches, and cough symptoms followed by rapid development of respiratory failure. Currently there have been 67 persons who have been affected, of these 22 were Navajos involving 12 deaths. At the outset of the Hantavirus Pulmonary Syndrome (HPS) the Navajo Nation Division of Health mobilized in coordination with the Navajo Area Indian Health Service, the three State Health Departments, University of New Mexico, CDC, and NIH to develop protocols and ascertain various medications to treat this illness.

As is the goals of the Navajo Division of Health is to manage a comprehensive health service which includes initiating a preventative community education program, coordination of a task force consisting of Navajo Nation Division of Health (DOH), Indian Health Service (IHS), & Centers for Disease Control (CDC), to begin clean up procedures, medical surveillance, seeking funds, and support of research to find answers to the Hantavirus that has affected the Navajo people as well as other regions of the United States. (ATTACHMENT A)

Attached is also the chronology of research activities done by Navajo Area Research and Publication Committee and Institutional Review Board (IRB) associated with human illness with the infections of the Hantavirus that has been identified in New Mexico, Colorado, Arizona, North Dakota,

Nevada, California and Texas. (ATTACHMENT B)

The Navajo Nation; Indian Health Service; University of New Mexico (UNM), National Institute of Health (NIH), and Centers for Disease Control (CDC), are continuing to wrestle with proposed medication study that will involve some Navajo families in the future, because the knowledge this new disease is extremely limited. Although Ribavirin is temporarily being administered on an experimental basis.

Let me reiterate the expeditious response that was implemented when the "Mysterious Illness" first occurred in the Four Corners area as Emergency was declared by the Navajo Nation; in collaboration with State Health Departments, Centers for Disease Control (CDC); University of New Mexico (UNM), and Indian Health Service (IHS). I would like to publicly commend all the key players such as Navajo Nation Health Education staff; Office of Environmental Health (OEH), Community Health Representative (CHR), Indian Health Service, Office of Environmental Health (IHS-OEH), University of New Mexico (UNM), Centers for Disease Control (CDC), National Institute of Health (NIH) for their untiring efforts to restore not only calmness but establish a final conclusion that the "deer mice" was the primary carrier of the HPS. Further, I would like to share with you some chronological events that occurred during this emergency.

1. Since June 04, 1993 Health Education operated Navajo Nation Hotline and NDOH, CDC, & FDA approved the compassionate use of Ribavirin drug.

2. June 08, 1993 Health Education staff conducted cultural awareness in service with CDC personnel.

3. In conjunction with WIC Media Specialist, the Winslow Health Education developed a poster on clean-up supplies and procedures.

4. Health Education/CHR's developed Navajo language video tape of the Hantavirus brochures to be disseminated to various media for prevention and education.

5. August 30, 1993, Health Educators, CHR's, OEH/NAIHS and PHN/NAIHS met to plan and formulate Hantavirus education and appropriate dissemination of information, clean up as the responsibility of the homeowners.

6. 10/93 - The NDOH in concert with NAIHS task force members developed (preliminary) Hantavirus clean up procedures and drafted a "Rodent Abatement Task Force for case homes."

   a. February and March 1994, the assessment of case homes were conducted and the Division of Health is in the process of obtaining materials and possible repair and replacement of materials that had to be removed due to rodent infestation.

   b. Thus far 15 case homes have been assessed and nine (9), more are pending.

7. Currently the NDOH and NAIHS have developed a protocol to respond to new confirmed cases of Hantavirus at the field level.

The Navajo Nation Division of Health and all relevant resources have and will continue to collaborate and coordinate their manpower and resources to insure that community education is imperative to promote prevention and awareness.

The Navajo Nation and Division of Health makes the following recommendations:

1. The Indian Health Service should maintain ALL their personnel to provide the necessary health care to Native Americans, more specifically, the Navajos.

2. No cuts should be allowed in the 121 projects but more funding to prevent any further Public Health crises as experienced and witnessed by the Nation the past year.

3. Congress and other elected officials shall be aware that the rural areas of America, especially reservations, like the Navajo Nation is extremely susceptible to Health crisis and are in need of Federal Funds to continue the health improvements of their populace.

4. Since there is direct relationship between the quality of health care and type of health/medical workers and adequacy of facilities, any reduction on IHS funding will have negative impact on the <u>level</u>, <u>quality</u>, and <u>coverage</u> of health services for the Navajo

Nation.

It is an honor and pleasure to present these concerns and problems before distinguished representatives and further appreciate continued cooperation and assistance that you and the Members of Congress can provide. Again, thank you.

Rodent Abatement Task Force

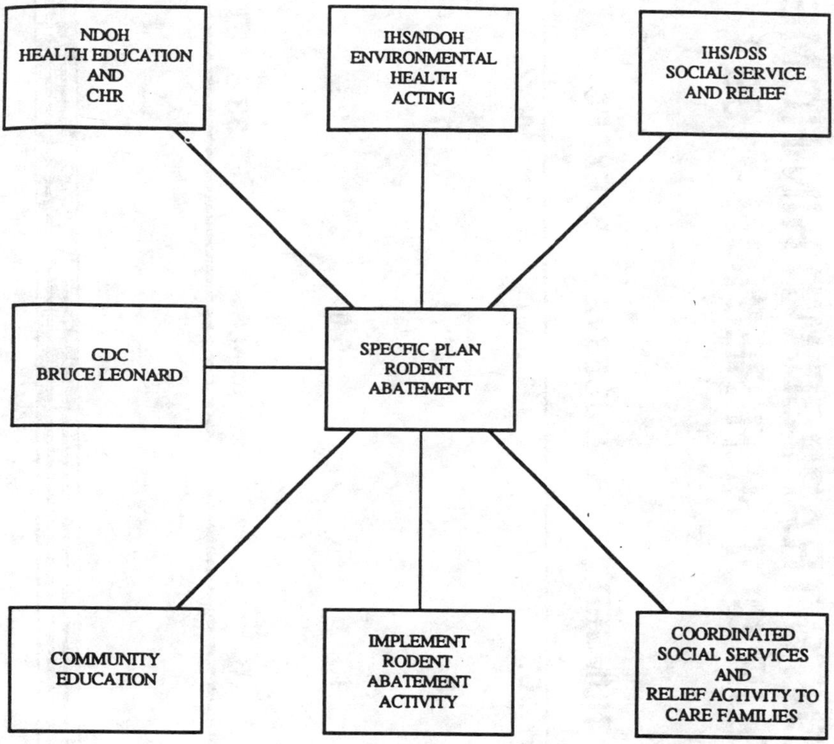

RODENTS TRAPPED WITHIN HOMES FOUR CORNER REGION - 1993

SPECIES	NUMBER	% OBSERVED	% EXPECTED
Peromyscus maniculatus	107	64.1	46.2
P. truei	34	20.4	17.6
Mus musculus	10	6.0	2.5
8 other species	16	9.6	33.8

CDC - DVRD - SPB

PREVALENCE OF PHV ANTIBODY FROM RODENTS CAPTURED WITHIN & OUTSIDE HUMAN DWELLINGS

	INSIDE		OUTSIDE	
RODENTS	POS.	NEG.	POS.	NEG.
Peromyscus (3 spp.)	48 (33.8)	94 (66.2)	295 (26.0)	838 (74.0)
OTHER SPECIES	3 (12.0)	22 (88.0)	17 (3.0)	546 (97.0)

CDC - DVRD - SPB

SPECIES COMPOSITION
FOUR CORNERS REGION

	N	%		N	%
Peromyscus maniculatus	770	45.4	*Neotoma albigula*	69	4.1
P. truei	314	18.5	*N. stephensi*	6	0.4
P. boylei	*59*	*3.5*	*N. mexicana*	20	1.2
Tamias dorsalis	156	9.2	*N. micropus*	4	0.2
T. quadrivittatus	46	2.7	*Cynomys gunnisoni*	1	0.1
T. minimus	12	0.7	*Dipodomys merriami*	4	0.2
Spermophilus variegatus	90	5.3	*D. ordii*	6	0.4
S. spilosoma	4	0.2	*Reithrodontomys megalotis*	9	0.5
S. lateralis	2	0.1	*Microtus longicaudus*	2	0.1
S. tridecemlineatus	7	0.4	*M. pennsylvanicus*	4	0.2
Mus musculus	56	3.3	*M. montanus*	2	0.1
Onychomys leucogaster	10	0.6	*Ammosperm. leucurus*	14	0.8

CDC - DVRD - SPB

SPECIES COMPOSITION
FOUR CORNERS REGION

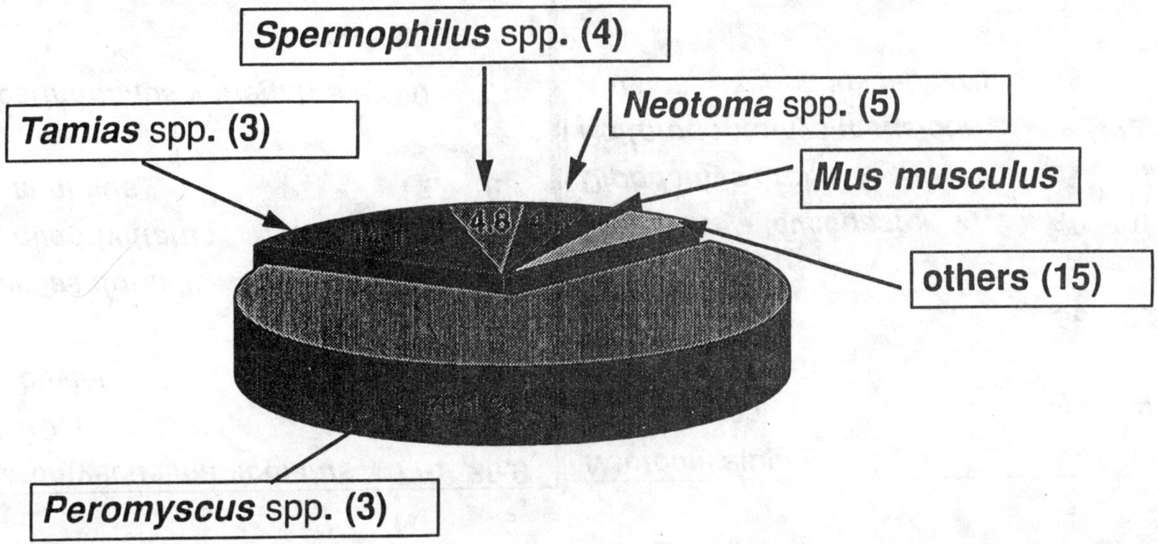

CDC - DVRD - SPB

PHV ANTIBODY PREVALENCE FOUR CORNERS REGION

	N	%
Peromyscus maniculatus	770	30.9
P. truei	314	19.7
P. boylei	59	6.8
Tamias dorsalis	156	2.6
T. quadrivittatus	46	15.2
T. minimus	12	0
Spermophilus variegatus	90	1.1

	N	%
Neotoma albigula	69	2.9
N. mexicana	20	0
Mus musculus	56	3.6
Onychomys leucogaster	10	0
Dipodomys ordii	6	0
Reithrodontomys megalotis	9	22.2
Ammospermophilus leucurus	14	0

CDC - DVRD - SPB

PHV ANTIBODY PREVALENCE BY LOCATION

LOCATION	RODENT Tested	RODENT Pos. (%)	*P. maniculatus* Tested	*P. maniculatus* Pos. (%)
New Mexico				
12 sites	957	16.5	386	29.3 (9.5-40.9)
Arizona				
6 sites	569	23.1	298	33.6 (23.9-37.4)
Colorado				
3 sites	172	19.0	86	29.1 (13.6-50.0)

CDC - DVRD - SPB

TRAPPING SCHEME
FOUR CORNERS REGION 1993

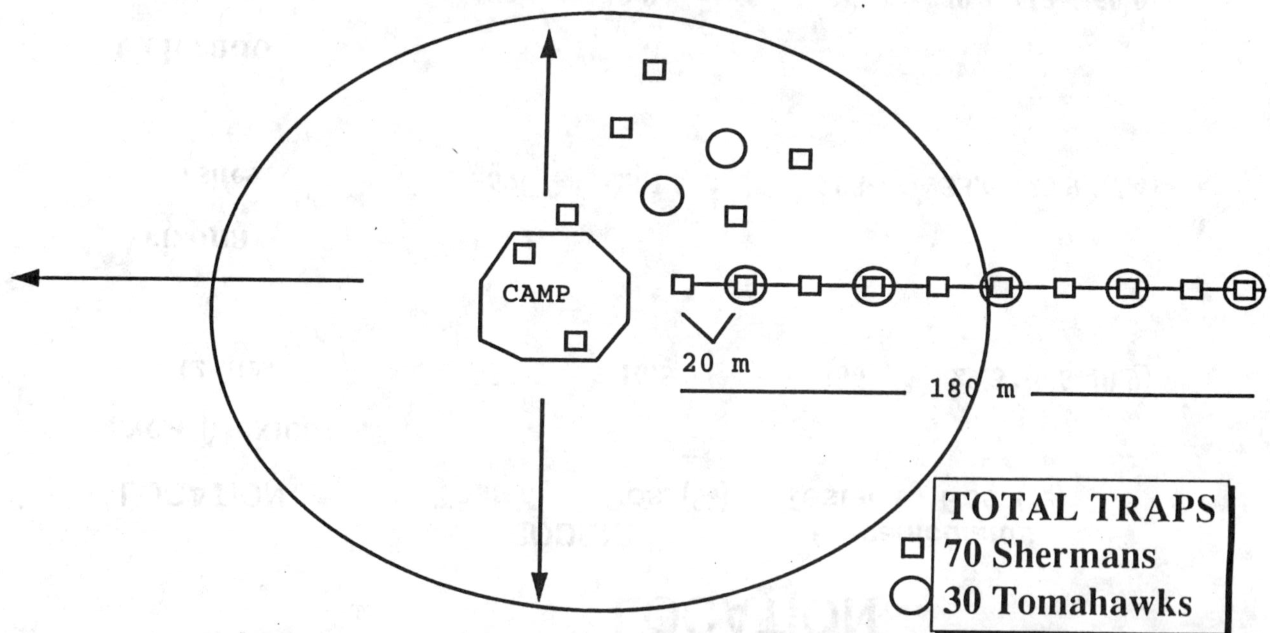

CDC - DVRD - SPB

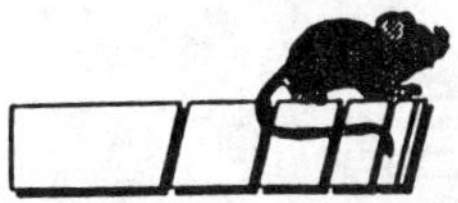

ADJUSTED TRAP SUCCESS
CASE & CONTROL HOUSES

LOCATION	CASE	CONTROL	RATIO
Crown Point	30.2	21.4	1.4
Ramah	40.7	31.5	1.3
IceCaves	49.1	22.3	2.2
Bread Springs	43.7	36.4	1.2
Vanderwagen	11.9	11.5	1.0
Hesperus	26.8	4.6	5.8
Farmington	0.0	0.0	---
Black Mesa	65.0	37.8	1.7
Jones Ranch	17.3	12.9	1.3
Sundance	16.9	12.7	1.3
Sedan	11.0	20.8	0.5
Grand Junction	5.1	14.4	0.4

CDC - DVRD - SPB

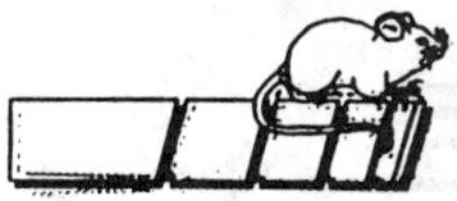

ADJUSTED TRAP SUCCESS (%) FOR CASE & CONTROL HOUSES

Case House	Near Control *	Far Control **
Greater than	18	13
Lesser than	4	4
Equal to	2	0

* P<0.005 Sign Test

** P<0.01 Sign Test

CDC - DVRD - SPB

NAVAJO AREA RESEARCH AND PUBLICATIONS COMMITTEE AND INSTITUTIONAL REVIEW BOARD (IRB)

ACTIVITIES RELATED TO HANTAVIRUS OUTBREAK

RESEARCH PROPOSALS

JUNE 7, 1993

REQUEST: Linda White
Chief, NAIHS Nutrition Branch

REQUEST BY CDC TO TEST EXISTING NUTRITION STUDY BLOOD SAMPLES FOR MYSTERY VIRUS (NAR-93-22)

DISPOSITION: Approved June 7 by Dr. Allen Craig, Acting Chairperson. Justification is CDC definition of "public health emergency" which grants the agency temporary exemption from IRB and OMB review and approval. Approval conditions: blood samples must be used anonymously, with only geographic area, age, and sex information provided. Approval granted only for this purpose. See NAR-93-13.

JUNE 8, 1993

REQUEST: Jay Butler, MD
Director, CDC Field Team

UNEXPLAINED ADULT RESPIRATORY DISTRESS SYNDROME (UARDS) OUTBREAK CASE CONTROL STUDY (NAR-93-13)

DISPOSITION: Approved June 8 by Acting Chairperson. Justification is CDC definition of "public health emergency." Approval noted that "standards of confidentiality, privacy, and security, required by 45 CFR 46, Protection of Human Subjects, particularly with regard to the informed consent process" should be observed. Also, (1) data are to be used only for purposes connected to the Hantavirus investigation, and (2) re-publication clearance of papers is requested. Papers which must be published quickly, e.g., in the CDC MMWR, will be handled expeditiously.

Agreement on July 2 with Lydia-Hubbard Pourier, Executive Director, Navajo Division of Health (and also an IRB member), and Donna Christensen, Navajo Nation legal counsel, requires that informed consent form be revised to include a statement regarding the possible need for future research on blood samples obtained during the survey.

JUNE 10, 1993

REQUEST: Louisa Chapman, MD
CDC Field Team

INTRAVENOUS RIBAVIRIN COMPASSIONATE USE REQUEST - UARDS OUTBREAK (NAR-93-14)

DISPOSITION: Approved June 10 by Acting Chairperson with concurrence by Lydia Hubbard-Pourier. Justification is (1) CDC definition of "public health emergency" and (2) "compassionate use" in the above emergency. Approval noted our expectation that "administration of Ribavirin will occur in accordance with all of the applicable provisions of 45 CFR 46, Protection of Human Subjects, regarding confidentiality and informed consent." Dr. Ray Reid, Committee member, is working with CDC representatives on the informed consent document. CDC also obtained the required approval from the Food and Drug Administration (FDA) for the use of Ribavirin as an "Investigational New Drug" (IND). See NAR-93-13.

<u>JUNE 18, 1993</u>

REQUEST: Mark Sawyer, MD (requested by Jay Butler)
University of California San Diego

AIR SAMPLING DEVICE - HANTAVIRUS OUTBREAK/CDC EPIDEMIOLOGICAL INVESTIGATION (NAR-93-21)

DISPOSITION: Approved June 23 by Acting Chairperson in consultation with Lydia Hubbard-Pourier. Justification is CDC definition of "public health emergency." Approval noted the following restrictions: (1) experimental equipment only to be used at rodent processing sites to monitor worker safety, (2) sensitivity to local community needs and concerns, (3) technology only to be used in connection with the CDC epidemiological investigation, and (4) pre-publication clearance of all papers. See NAR-93-13.

<u>JUNE 21, 1993</u>

REQUEST: James McLaughlin, PhD
Director, Microbiology Lab
University of New Mexico Hospital

REQUEST FROM UNIVERSITY OF NEW MEXICO HOSPITAL TO USE PATIENT LAB SPECIMENS FOR HANTAVIRUS RAPID DIAGNOSTIC TEST (NAR-93-27)

DISPOSITION: Agreement reached July 2 by Acting Chairperson in consultation with Lydia Hubbard-Pourier and Donna Christensen, Navajo Nation legal counsel. Conference call on 6/24 to discuss immediate use of existing specimens as well as access to other specimens, including CDC and others. Guidelines needed because the National Institutes of Health (NIH) is soon to release monies for Hantavirus research. Technically, we have no jurisdiction over existing UNM hospital specimens; this is a courtesy request. But other requests are sure to follow, which we will be asked to review and approve. Cultural/spiritual issues, regarding proper handling and disposal of blood, urine, and tissue samples, have been raised by committee member Ray Reid, a Navajo physician, as well as others. UNM has asked for a meeting to establish some guidance. Representatives from CDC, New Mexico Office of the Medical Investigator, and others want to be included.

Agreement includes following points: (1) only applies to existing lab specimens, (2) further analysis for purpose of developing rapid diagnostic test, (3) handle specimens in accordance with 45 CFR 46, as determined by UNM IRB, and (4) handle reports for publication with care and sensitivity.

JUNE 28, 1993

REQUEST: Mary Jane Schmidt, MD, and Lone Simonsen, PhD (transmitted by Rick Haskins) CDC Field Team

OUTBREAK OF UNEXPLAINED ARDS IN FOUR CORNERS AREA: FOLLOW-UP CASES WITH PRODROMAL-LIKE ILLNESS (NAR-93-25)

DISPOSITION: Considered approved (July 1) as part of CDC Hantavirus epidemiological investigation. Revised informed consent form required. See NAR-93-13.

JULY 2, 1993

REQUEST: C. Vitek, Rob Breiman, MD, F. Foster, Edith Umland, MD, and UARDS Study Task Force

HOSPITAL CONTACTS OF PATIENTS WITH UARDS STUDY PROTOCOL (NAR-93-30)

DISPOSITION: Considered approved (July 2) as part of CDC Hantavirus epidemiological investigation. Revised informed consent form required. See NAR-93-13.

JULY 6, 1993

REQUEST: Ron Moolenaar, MD, Jeff Duchin, MD, Edith Umland, MD, Rob Breiman, MD, and UARDS Study Task Force

IDENTIFICATION OF CLINICAL FACTORS ASSOCIATED WITH HANTA-LIKE VIRUS INFECTION (NAR-93-32)

DISPOSITION: Considered approved (July 6) as part of CDC Hantavirus epidemiological investigation. See NAR-93-13.

JULY 27, 1993

REQUEST: C. Vitek and UARDS Study Task Force

SEROPREVALENCE OF HANTAVIRUS IN IHS ENVIRONMENTAL HEALTH PROFESSIONALS PROTOCOL (NAR-93-35)

DISPOSITION: Considered approved (July 29) as part of CDC Hantavirus epidemiological investigation. See NAR-93-13.

AUGUST 25, 1993

REQUEST: B. Muneta and UARDS Study Task Force

EVALUATION OF FOUR CORNERS HEALTH EDUCATION PROJECT (NAR-93-40)

DISPOSITION: Full IRB review. Approved (8/31/93) as Navajo Nation project.

PUBLICATIONS

NOT REVIEWED

KOSTER, F. AND OTHERS
1993 **Outbreak of Acute Illness - Southwestern US, 1993.** CDC Mortality/Morbidity Weekly Report (MMWR), June 11.

KOSTER, F. AND OTHERS
1993 **Update: Outbreak of Hantavirus Infection - Southwestern US, 1993.** CDC Mortality/Morbidity Weekly Report (MMWR), June 18.

KOSTER, F. AND OTHERS
1993 **Update: Outbreak of Hantavirus Infection - Southwestern US, 1993.** CDC Mortality/Morbidity Weekly Report (MMWR), June 25.

KOSTER, F. AND OTHERS
1993 **Update: Outbreak of Hantavirus Infection - Southwestern US, 1993.** CDC Mortality/Morbidity Weekly Report (MMWR), July 1.

KOSTER, F. AND OTHERS
1993 **Update: Outbreak of Hantavirus Infection - Southwestern US, 1993.** CDC Mortality/Morbidity Weekly Report (MMWR), July 9.

CDC
1993 **Hantavirus Infection - Southwestern United States: Interim Recommendations for Risk Reduction.** CDC Mortality/Morbidity Weekly Report (MMWR), August 30.

EXPEDITED REVIEW/APPROVAL

NICHOL, S. AND OTHERS
1993 **Genetic Identification of a Novel Hantavirus Associated with an Outbreak of Acute Respiratory Illness in the Southwestern United States.** To be published in the journal *Science*.

ABSTRACT

CHAPMAN, L. AND OTHERS
1993 **Investigational Intravenous Ribavirin in US Hantavirus Infections.**

REVISED 10/19/93

NAVAJO NATION TESTIMONY
HEALTH CARE FACILITIES AND SANITATION FACILITIES PROJECTS

Mr. Chairman and members of the Subcommittee, I am Peggy Nakai, Health Program Manager of the Office of Special Projects for the Navajo Division of Health. I appreciate the opportunity and am honored to present the Navajo Nation's views and recommendations on the IHS budget cuts particularly concerning proposed Navajo Area IHS hospitals and clinics and sanitation facilities (waterline projects). We look forward to working with your Subcommittee on these two issues.

The Navajo Nation has a total population of 212,343 with approximately 195,470 residing on the reservation. As a Nation we are the largest Native American Indian tribe and granted we are respected for the progress that we have made in tribal policy and infrastructure development. However, there are many things which still need work. Today, the Navajo people are still struggling to attain the things which the rest of the American society have taken for granted such as indoor plumbing, running water, electricity, telephones, paved roads, washing machines, adequate housing, accessible shopping centers and good medical care. The list goes on and on.

FACILITIES (HOSPITALS AND CLINICS DESIGN/CONSTRUCTION)
For the past twenty years, the Navajo Nation has been actively requesting Congress and the Indian Health Service to replace the SHIPROCK HOSPITAL, build a new health center at TOHATCHI, both of which are in New Mexico and replace the FORT DEFIANCE HOSPITAL in Arizona. The Navajo Nation is proud to state the fact that the Navajo Area Indian Health Service is only one of a few IHS Areas across the United States which provides much of the primary health care services to its Native American population, while many of the other Areas contract with private providers for their medical care. The Navajo Nation does not have immediate plans to begin contracting with private providers for its medical care services. As a Nation, we plan to continue supporting and advocating for improvement and replacement of IHS Hospitals and Clinics. Over the years, there has been much time, resources and manpower expended by the Navajo Nation in lobbying and planning for these facilities inspite of the many setbacks, policy changes, changes in administrations and changes in appropriations policies that have occurred.

SHIPROCK HOSPITAL
As you know, there is a beautiful new IHS hospital about 75% complete under construction at this time here in SHIPROCK and the design for the hospital won a national design award. However, the FY1995 IHS Budget cuts have resulted in the very real possibility of opening the new $57 Million facility with only a fraction of the total number of staff needed to operate at optimum capacity. The user population for the new facility is approximately 45,000 people within the Four Corners area. There are 21 Navajo chapters in the Shiprock Service Unit area. The new 215,826 square foot hospital

requires 515 additional staff at a cost of $23,610,175, including an additional $9.2 Million for activation expenses. Without these funds, some of the specialty services and operational funds will be eliminated which will negatively impact on the overall provision of health care services. The patient waiting times will increase and there will be more referrals to off-reservation medical providers.

TOHATCHI HEALTH CENTER
As a result of the proposed FTE cuts in the FY1995 IHS Budget, Congress must restore approximately $3,354,000 needed to hire 63 additional staff to operate the new TOHATCHI health center at optimum levels. The new 38,000 square foot health center is scheduled for completion early this summer and will serve five nearby communities, as well as accommodate some of the patient overflow during the renovation of the Gallup Indian Medical Center scheduled to begin this summer. The scheduled renovation is expected to last approximately 14 months.

FORT DEFIANCE HOSPITAL
The Navajo Nation is requesting first phase construction funds for the new FORT DEFIANCE HOSPITAL in the amount of $37 Million to initiate the construction phase upon completion of the design in FY 1995. However, the IHS budget did not include a request in its FY 1995 Budget for the first phase construction funds. If it is not feasible to fund this request at the maximum level, then the construction funds must be further broken down into smaller incremental allocations over the next four fiscal years. The Navajo Nation would then respectfully request approximately $5.1 million to conduct the site work and utilities for the first phase. The second phase will require an additional $8.6 million to continue to complete the site work, utilities and foundation work. The third phase requires approximately $14.2 million for the site work, utilities, foundation and super structure. The final phase requires $20.0 million for the enclosed building. For a total cost of $48 Million.

RED MESA HEALTH CENTER
The Navajo Nation is awaiting final approval of the proposed planning documents (Program Of Requirements and Program Justification Documents) by the IHS Headquarters. Recently, an analysis was requested by the IHS Headquarters regarding the feasibility of instituting the utilization of two facilities to serve the Utah Navajos. The Navajo Nation is supportive of this proposal but requests that a more centrally located satellite facility be considered so that accessibility is assured to those Navajos living in the bordertowns off-reservation. Further, an expeditious review and approval is requested.

DILKON HEALTH CENTER
The Navajo Nation requests a replacement facility for the Winslow Health Center. The Dilkon community is requesting an appropriation from Congress in the amount of $20 Million to design and construct a new health facility which would replace the Winslow Health Center. The Winslow Health Center was ordered condemned after the

1971 earthquake, however, the Navajo Area Indian Health Service closed the inpatient unit and continued to provide health care services in its outpatient department. Recently, another structural assessment was conducted by Bacchus Engineering, of Albuquerque, New Mexico, whose report recommended the building be demolished as soon as practicable.

STAFF QUARTERS

An adequate number of staff quarters is essential to retaining and recruiting qualified medical staff. Medical staff are required to be available on a 24 hour basis to assure provision of essential medical services; this requires an adequate number of staff quarters to be made more readily available. Currently in the Navajo Area, housing is not available for sale or rent anywhere on the Reservation. Lack of adequate housing near the medical facilities means that some staff are travelling one or two hours a day to get to and from work. Eventually, the constant travel begins to take its toll on people. Often, family relationships become strained because of the constant hours away from family activities. On the job, there is more absenteeism, sickness and fatigue. Gradually, staff begin to look for employment and move to places where there is easier and greater accessibility to their jobs, shopping and entertainment.

SAFE WATER AND SANITARY WASTE DISPOSAL FACILITIES (P.L. 86-121 Projects)

The Navajo Nation requests a complete restoration of the $85,272,000 to the FY 1995 IHS Budget for sanitation facilities. Of the $85,272,000, approximately $25 Million was requested for expanding waterlines for about 500 Navajo families. According to the 1990 Census, approximately 51% of the Navajo Reservation homes lack indoor plumbing. There is still a great deal of work needed to be done.

The American society lives in a technologically advanced society. All over the world, people dream of coming to live in America. Yet today in Washington D.C.'s own backyard, Native American people are hauling water to drink, bathe and water their livestock as often as once a week. In some places on the reservation, people must drive 50-60 miles round trip to the nearest water source.

In the healthcare profession, the emphasis is prevention. Much of the health promotion activities stress cleanliness. However, cleanliness must take a backseat to preservation of this precious commodity for drinking water. Lack of adequate water prohibits those with medical problems to follow the doctor's orders and recommendations to sustain their health or to improve their health conditions. Diabetics have a particularly difficult time maintaining their diets and ensuring that their feet are healthy and free of sores, when they do not have an adequate water supply.

In the Health Care Improvement Act Section 302. subsection (a) Congress finds and declares that-- and I quote:

"(1) the provision of safe water supply systems and sanitary sewage and solid waste disposal systems is primarily a health consideration and function;

(2) Indian people suffer an inordinately high incidence of disease, injury, and illness directly attributable to the absence or inadequacy of such systems;

(3) the long-term cost to the United States of treating and curing such disease, injury, and illness is substantially greater than the short-term cost of providing such systems and other preventive health measures;

(4) many Indian homes and communities still lack safe water supply systems and sanitary sewage and solid waste disposal systems; and

(5) it is in the interest of the United States, and it is the policy of the United States, that all Indian communities and Indian homes, new and existing, be provided with safe and adequate water supply systems and sanitary sewage and solid waste disposal systems as soon as possible."

I read this portion of the Health Care Improvement Act to remind us of what Congress has agreed to provide to Native Americans. As stated in the Federal Act, the government is obligated because of its treaty obligations and responsibilities to ensure that all Native Americans receive adequate funds and assistance to improve their health status.

I've often heard the comment from the Indian Health Service when they are attempting to seek third party payment for services, "if only the tribe would pay", I am reminded that our forefathers have already paid a GREAT price. As you travel across this great land, you will also remember that a great price has already been paid. Yes, these services are not "free", they have been paid for by our ancestors prior to receipt of services!!

NAVAJO NATION TESTIMONY ON TEEN HEALTH

The Navajo population is a very young population, 50% being under the age of 18 (approximately one-third of the total Navajo population is between the ages of 12 and 20). As such, the current health status and well being of Navajo youth is crucial to the welfare, survival and continued progress of the Navajo Nation. Navajo parents, educators, tribal officials, public safety officials, health care providers, and community workers are not very happy with the health status of the today's Navajo youth. Furthermore, they have noticed a wide discrepancy in the health care services and resources needed by Navajo youth and what is already available for them. Compared to youth from the rest of the country, Navajo youth come from a much poorer and different home background (both socially and economically), they live in poorer sanitary conditions, they have to travel long distances to access educational and medical facilities and they have hardly any recreational facilities to keep them occupied during the weekends and summer time. All these have lead to a low spiritual, mental, emotional, and physical health for the Navajo youth. However, up-to-date and precise statistics on health care issues concerning Navajo youth are currently lacking. Current studies underway on the reservation should shed some light on the matter, which in turn could be used to improve the current health status of Navajo youth.

The picture of Navajo health is not very easy to draw. For the Navajo, like other Native Americans, health goes beyond physical health. The total picture of health is a culmination of physical, spiritual, emotional, mental and environmental health. It is the health of the individuals, the family unit, the clan and the whole nation. It ascends from the home to the grass roots level to the chapter and to the whole nation. Progress, on one hand, has brought many materialistic comforts to the Navajo people, but in the struggle to "fit in", the Navajo and especially the youth, are torn between their roots and the ways of modern (white) society. Education and health care services available (even if inadequate) have improved the basic physical health status of the Navajo youth, but the added pressure brought in by the need to "succeed" in today's society has made it necessary for many to give up their language, belief system, religion , and culture, and become "assimilated" into the larger society. The addiction to sugar, salt, and fat has lead to obesity. A sedentary life at school away from taking care of "chores" at home has led the youth away from the traditional active and health lifestyle. They have been forced to change their philosophy from taking care of things for now to think about the future. Especially for those youth hailing from traditional homes, these stressful situations have been too much to handle. The consequence: the leading cause of the death for the Navajo youth today is accidents, stemming from the alcohol use related incidents, whether related to vehicle use or pedestrian traffic, getting into fights, disruptive behaviors, sexual activity, or self-inflicted injury (planned or accidental). Tormented by boredom and depression leading from inability to cope or problems arising from dysfunctional families, the young people are turning to alcohol and drugs at an earlier age, and as the years go by, the severity of substance abuse is increasing. Leading causes of substance abuse related injury and deaths include motor vehicle-passenger accidents, motor vehicle-pedestrian accidents, fires/burns, drowning, suicides, and homicides. Many of these numbers seem to be alarmingly high for the Navajo male adolescents. The patient load for the Indian Health Service being high, the lack of easy accessibility to the facilities, the fast turn over of health care providers, and the delay in the delivery system all make the matters even worse. It may not be difficult, with enough funds and trained manpower, to document these conditions; but it is not enough to just have quantitative data. It is more important to have qualitative data available to understand and comprehend the true health status of Navajo youth.

The lack of or inadequate parental involvement in the health and welfare of the youth is a common outcry in this country, but on the Reservation, one needs to wonder whether the problem arises from the lack of parental involvement or the inability of parents to be involved. This inability may stem from lack of formal education, language barrier, and/or implementation of services alien to the Navajo way. More and more, the IHS has modeled services t fit the unique needs of the Navajo but somehow, the basic health education which needs to go with these services does not seem to have filtered into the homes. Once a unique and workable system of parental education is in place, we could surely expect a change in the health status of the Navajo . This means ignorance and alienation should be removed and replaced by knowledge and acceptance.

NAVAJO NATION TESTIMONY ON WOMEN'S HEALTH ISSUES

The general overall health status of the Native American Indian population is integrally tied to the health status of the Indian women. Although improvements have been made in the area of maternal and infant mortality, the health status of Indian women is far from optimal. Indian women suffer disproportionately from lifestyle related diseases and premature deaths. Significant health issues among Indian women which the IHS and tribes needs more funding to address are:

1. Cancer
2. Diabetes
3. OB/GYN issues
4. Alcoholism/Substance Abuse
5. Pyschosocial Issues
6. Family Violence
7. Research
8. Elderly Issues
9. Access to care

The New Mexico Tumor registry for example indicates that Indian women with cancer are diagnosed at a more advanced stage and their survival is much worse than non-Indian women. IHS must develop its capacity for early detection and patient care for all preventable diseases like breast and cervical cancers.

Navajo society is a matrilineal order based on kinship. Navajo women are the center of the home and their role is very important to the preservation of the Navajo culture and society. It is through the Navajo woman that the clan or kinship is traced which identifies every Navajo child. This identity creates unity among the Navajo people and everyone is considered family. The Navajo woman takes the primary responsibility for making the important decisions about all of the issues pertaining to the maintenance, sustenance and nurturance of the members residing therein. Like the dominant society, however, divorce has taken its toll on Navajo families. There are many single parent homes where Navajo mothers assume a dual role of breadwinner and nurturer for the family, often resulting in poor health due to lack of adequate health care services.

Navajo women residing on the Navajo reservation have a tendency to be very modest and inhibited by traditional taboos, which affects the acceptance of the Western medicine, participate in self-exams, and to seek preventive health education information. There is a definite language barrier between the medical provider and the patient, especially the Navajo elderly women. Linguistically speaking, there are many diseases which are not translatable into Navajo. Interpretation and translation of the technical medical language becomes very difficult and sometimes the meaning is lost which prohibits the patient from fully understanding the circumstance of her disease. Also, terminal illness or potential death is not discussed because it is taboo to discuss one's life in those terms.

More funds are also needed to augment the outreach health services programs for the rural and underserved Indian women especially for screening and early detection of many preventable diseases.

Cultural barriers have contributed to under-utilization of medical care. Modesty, taboos, and utilization of traditional healing practices are important elements of a cultural belief system maintained among the Navajo. Beliefs about modern medical procedures for detecting and treating diseases like breast and cervical cancers may also be barriers.

Many of the reservation residents have suffered from disintegration of the family unit, high unemployment rates, serious behavioral and emotional problems, and morbidity and mortality rates which are more than double those of the general population.

According to the Navajo Area Status by Life Stages, the leading causes of death for Navajo adult women ages 20 through 44 years are in this order:

-- Accidents, Adverse Effects (including Motor Vehicle)
-- Chronic Liver Disease/Cirrhosis
-- Suicide
-- Heart Disease
-- Neoplasms (cancer)

The leading causes of death for Navajo women aged 45 and over are:

-- Neoplasms
-- Heart Disease
-- Diabetes
-- Accidents, Adverse Effects (including Motor Vehicle)

The following recommendations are made:

1. The Navajo Nation and the IHS need to work together to develop policies, planning and services to meet the health care needs of the underserved Navajo female population.

2. Since Diabetes ranks in the top ten leading causes of the death of the American Indian/Alaskan Natives, the IHS and tribes need to focus on programs which have succeeded in curbing this disease, to share the information and implement. Renal Dialysis needs to be more easily accessible so that diabetics can enjoy a better quality of life.

3. More research monies for development of qualitative data on diseases impacting Native American women is needed.

TESTIMONY
for
Senators McCain and Domenici

Navajo Nation AIDS Office

Honorable Senators McCain and Domenici, Honorable Navajo Nation President Zah, Honorable Councilwoman Genevieve Jackson, distinguished guest, ladies and gentlemen, and Navajo Nation staff, I am honored and grateful to present the status of AIDS epidemic on the Navajo Nation and programmatic efforts to combat this devastating disease.

Historically, the Navajo Nation as a people have suffered adversities of health-related epidemics such as Tuberculosis, Hepatitis and other communicable diseases that have afflicted the Navajo people in major outbreaks.

AIDS, an incurable disease that has confronted the society worldwide is rapidly and dangerously soaring among the Native Americans and Alaska Natives, including the Navajo people. The background for considering what it will take to prevent and control AIDS involves both the current status of the pandemic and the status of the Navajo Nation's response.

As of January 1993, more than half a million AIDS cases had been officially reported to the World Health Organization; a yet more realistic estimate by the World Health Organization is that AIDS has developed in nearly 3 million adults and more than 750,000 children since the beginning of the pandemic.

Among the Native Americans and Alaska Natives, according to the IHS Headquarters West, as of September 1993, reported there were 731 reported AIDS cases, 301 cases of which were from the Southwest Region. The Navajo Nation occupies three southwest states. More specifically, the Navajo Area IHS reported 49 cumulative AIDS cases or about 20 percent of the Southwest Region, of which 16 are deceased, 29 are HIV-positive, and 4 are living with AIDS. It is estimated that the numbers are remarkably higher resulting from under-reporting, underdiagnosis, and delay in reporting. In addition, these numbers reflect only those Navajo individuals seen by IHS or at facilities paid for by IHS. It does not represent those Navajo individuals seeking HIV services outside the IHS system or have not been tested.

More importantly, the National AIDS Coordinator further reported that the percentage of American Indian and Alaska Native women of child bearing age with HIV was 4 to 8 times higher that of women in the general population. On the Navajo Nation, 16 percent of the known HIV/AIDS cases reported are female.

What is more frightening is the recent information published by the Centers for Disease Control and Prevention documented that 82 percent increase in the number of persons between the ages of 13-19 were counseled and tested for HIV between 1991 and 1992, and most significant rate of increase in diagnosed AIDS cases has occurred among the 20-24 age group. Due to the known median incubation period between HIV infection and AIDS diagnosis is about 10 years, it is clear that a significant number of those individuals in their twenties who are diagnosed with AIDS were teenagers when they became infected. The IHS Headquarters West quarterly report of November 29, 1993 is included at **Attachment A**

Until medical research finds a cure for AIDS, we must rely on changes in personal behavior to stop the spread of HIV. Therefore, an effective AIDS education and prevention activities are vital. The Navajo Nation has assumed leadership to educate the Navajo people regarding the dangers of HIV and AIDS through its AIDS Office and through networking with community-based organizations on AIDS, tribal programs and IHS.

The Navajo Nation Council understands the devastating effects of HIV, and realizes the adverse impact of the increased rate of HIV cases on the Navajo Nation. In order to confine the prevalence of HIV and AIDS not to exceed the national average among the Native Americans and Alaska Natives, the Navajo Nation Council, in March 1993, appropriated tribal funds to create an AIDS Office. Although the AIDS Office was opened with a traditional blessing, in March 1993, the program actually commenced in September 1993.

The Navajo Nation AIDS Office functions under the auspices of the Executive Director, Navajo Division of Health, and is staffed with four positions. The primary responsibility of the Navajo Nation AIDS Office is to provide culturally appropriate AIDS education, and coordinate AIDS prevention activities with community-based organizations on AIDS. Currently, the AIDS Office is overwhelmed with requests from schools for AIDS prevention activities as proms and graduations are rapidly approaching. Further, the AIDS Office is involved in the planning of alcohol and drug free prom and graduation dances with various schools.

The Navajo Nation AIDS Policy Development Work Group, a sub-committee of the Health and Social Services Committee of the Navajo Nation Council-an oversight committee of the divisions of health and social services, is comprised of members of the Health and Social Services Committee, community-based organizations on AIDS, and representatives from various tribal programs, including the Occupational Safety and Health, the STD Control Program, the Office of Chief Justice, and the Navajo Nation AIDS Office provides support staff to the work group. The work group have been convening approximately two years and the fruit of their labor is a proposed Navajo Nation AIDS Policy. The policy is currently undergoing a legislative review. It is anticipated that the proposed policy will be presented before the Navajo Nation Council for enactment during its spring session. When enacted, the Navajo Nation AIDS Policy will mandate that AIDS be a top priority in an effort to stop the spread on the Navajo Nation, and it will guide all tribal programs, health care providers and businesses to provide education, counseling, compassion, and to protect individuals from discrimination or invasion of privacy. <u>The proposed Navajo Nation AIDS Policy is included at **Attachment B**</u>.

In collaboration with the Navajo Nation Council on Aging, the AIDS Office has trained ten Navajo foster grandparents on HIV and AIDS. The foster grandparents are committed and dedicated to providing AIDS education that is consistent and acceptable to the traditional practices and customs of the Navajo Nation.

The Navajo Nation AIDS Office intends to continue utilizing the Navajo elderly in providing AIDS education and enhance its network with community-based organizations, IHS, states and other health organizations.

Although the Navajo Division of Health is pursuing to contract an AIDS prevention program from the Navajo Area IHS pursuant to P.L. 93-638, it will provide limited staff and travel support which will not adequately fund the AIDS Office to implement AIDS education throughout the Navajo Nation.

Therefore, the Navajo Nation AIDS Office is urging the Honorable Senators and Representative to mandate all schools operating on the Navajo Nation and in border towns attended by the Navajo students, particularly state-funded schools to include AIDS education in educational curricula, and to mandate the Department of Education to include staff and travel support to implement AIDS education and prevention activities.

In the future, I hope the State Legislature will continue to support prevention activities against the spread of AIDS and allow Native Americans to participate on other health endeavors.

The Navajo Nation AIDS Office is applaud to be included in this hearing that could allow for an increase and expansion of the AIDS prevention activities throughout the Navajo Nation. Thank you for the opportunity to speak before you.

Attachment "A"

DEPARTMENT OF HEALTH & HUMAN SERVICES

Memora

Date 29 November 1993

From Area AIDS Coordinator
NAIHS

Subject HIV/AIDS Cases on Navajo

To Emmett Chase, M.D., M.P.H.
National Coordinator
AIDS Activities Office, IHS HQ West

The following data currently reflects the HIV disease affecting the Navajo

49 Cumulative Total (two individuals are not Navajo but are Native
41 males (First Case on Navajo was in 1982)
8 females
16 deaths
4 living with AIDS
29 HIV infected

This data is further delineated to show age and sex of those infected.

Under 20		20-24		30-34		40+	
3		16		17		13	
M	F	M	F	M	F	M	F
2	1	14	2	14	3	11	2

Mode of transmission data is unavailable since many of the cases are deemc
unknown by the patients themselves.

If you have any questions, please call (505) 368-2480.

Chris Percy, M.D.

REPORTED CASES OF AIDS IN AMERICAN INDIANS AND ALASKA NATIVES

As of September 30, 1993
Date

1. The number of American Indians and Alaska Natives (AI/AN) with AIDS 731
2. The number of these that are male 623
3. The number under 13 years of age at the time of first diagnosis 14
4. The number that have died 354 (Adult/adolescent) 10 (Peds (<13 years old))
5. Age range: 0 to 72 Mean age: 34
6. **Age at Diagnosis:**

	Number	%
Under 5	13	1.8
5 - 12	1	0.1
13 - 19	12	1.6
20 - 29	179	24.5
30 - 39	347	47.5
40 - 49	133	18.2
Over 49	46	6.3

7. **Transmission Categories for Adults/Adolescents:**

	Number	% of adult cases
Men who have sex with men	338	54.11
Injecting drug use (female & heterosexual male)	114	15.90
Men who have sex with men and inject drugs	107	14.92
Hemophilia/coagulation disorder	16	2.23
Heterosexual cases	42	5.86
Transfusion, blood components	13	1.81
Undetermined	37	5.16

Transmission Categories for Children (<13 years old):

	Number	% of pediatric cases
Hemophilia/coagulation disorder	1	7.14
Mother with/at risk of HIV infection	13	92.86
Transfusion, blood components	0	
Undetermined	0	

8. Opportunistic Disease Category:

	Number	%
Pneumocystis carinii pneumonia	289	39.5
Kaposi's sarcoma	74	10.1
PCP and KS	26	3.6
Other opportunistic diseases (excl. PCP & KS)	381	52.1

9. Cases of AIDS in Native Americans & All U.S. Races by Year of Report & Diagnosis

	Number Entered at CDC		Number Diagnosed	
Year	AI/AN	All Races including AI/AN	AI/AN	All Races including AI/AN
Before 1983	2	831	2	1,563
1983	0	2093	0	3,040
1984	3	4503	5	6,102
1985	10	8290	12	11,576
1986	20	13237	29	18,766
1987	29	21245	39	28,164
1988	40	31929	60	34,857
1989	71	35031	77	41,215
1990	85	43282	102	45,491
1991	88	45388	131	53,861
1992	115	47224	188	62,804
1993	268	86,197	86	31,811

10. The number of cases according to Starcher-defined regions:

	Number	
Southwest:	301	Arizona, California, Colorado, Guam, Hawaii, Nevada, New Mexico, Trust Territory, Utah.
Northwest:	98	Alaska, Idaho, Montana, Oregon, Washington, Wyoming.
Midwest:	215	Arkansas, Illinois, Indiana, Iowa, Kansas, Louisiana, Michigan, Minnesota, Missouri, Nebraska, North Dakota, Ohio, Oklahoma, South Dakota, Texas, Wisconsin.
Northeast:	69	Connecticut, Delaware, Maine, Maryland, Massachusetts, New Hampshire, New Jersey, New York, Pennsylvania, Rhode Island, Vermont, District of Columbia.
Southeast:	48	Alabama, Florida, Georgia, Kentucky, Mississippi, North Carolina, Puerto Rico, South Carolina, Tennessee, Virgin Islands, Virginia, West Virginia.

78-786 - 94 - 9

Proposed

NAVAJO NATION AIDS POLICY STATEMENT

Prepared by:

THE NAVAJO NATION AIDS POLICY DEVELOPMENT COMMITTEE

Harry Hubbard, Health & Social Services Committee
Navajo Nation Council

Melvin Harrison, President, Navajo Nation AIDS Network
John Wilson, Navajo Nation AIDS Network

Paul George, Director,
Navajo Occupational Safety & Health Administration

Roselyn Chapela, Manager
Navajo Nation AIDS Office

Larry P. Foster, Social Hygiene Specialist
Navajo Nation Division of Health

Al Harris, Supreme Court Law Clerk
Navajo Nation Supreme Court

Dan Vicenti, Deputy Director of Judicial Administration
Navajo Nation Judicial Branch

January 12, 1994
Window Rock, Navajo Nation (Arizona)

NAVAJO NATION AIDS POLICY STATEMENT

Introduction

The Navajo Nation[1] issues this AIDS Policy Statement (Policy Statement) to address various issues as a result of the rise in the number of acquired immune deficiency syndrome (AIDS)[2] cases among its people and realizing the potential catastrophic impact of AIDS.

The Policy Statement is founded primarily on Navajo culture and Navajo history. The past demonstrates that Navajos can prevail over adversities and obstacles. A strong, comprehensive kinship system compelling solidarity is a strength of the Navajo people and a major reason for Navajo survival. The Policy Statement, therefore, reflects compassion in the broader Navajo value of *K'e*[3].

---

[1] The Navajo Nation includes tribal trust land, the "Checkerboard Area", the New Lands, and the satellite reservation communities of Ramah, Alamo, and Canoncito, New Mexico.

[2] The term "AIDS" is used in this Policy Statement to refer to all persons infected by human immunodeficiency virus (HIV). HIV-infected (seropositive) and fully diagnosed Acquired Immunodeficiency Syndrome. "HIV-infected" means seropositive or testing positively to HIV virus, but showing no signs of illness.

[3] "K'e" is a Navajo word meaning relationship. It can be used to mean biological or clan descent relation relationships and groups of relatives. Through k'e, the Navajo people know one another and how to act appropriately towards each other. K'e defines the Navajo's relationship with all other beings and forces in the universe. "K'e" (according to translation by Witherspoon, 1975, p. 37) translates into English as compassion, cooperation, friendliness, unselfishness, peacefulness, and all those positive

The right of each person to be respected as a unique individual is the focus of the Policy Statement. It incorporates the right of a person to be free from discrimination and unfair treatment, including harassment, due to infection or a perception that the person may or could be infected or a carrier. Finally, the Policy Statement is based on the belief that every citizen of the Navajo Nation has the right to receive health care and medical treatment for HIV/AIDS.

AIDS is a Health Problem Affecting the Navajo Nation

HIV/AIDS is not only a city problem; it is now a health problem affecting the Navajo Nation. Navajo Nation leaders must recognize AIDS as a devastating disease, because of the severity of the sickness involved. A person can contract HIV or AIDS on the reservation or in most any off-reservation community where he or she assumes or is subjected to the risk. People infected with HIV/AIDS often suffer rejection, persecution, and mistreatment.

There is no risk to others if a person contracts AIDS or is infected with the AIDS virus (HIV), unless an uninfected person has unprotected sex with an infected person without taking precautions[4], or unless the uninfected person shares contaminated

values which create an intense, diffuse, and enduring solidarity.

[4] Safer sex precautions include not having sexual intercourse without use of a latex condom; not having oral intercourse; and not sharing sex toys that have been used by anyone else.

needles. The risk of contracting HIV or AIDS is greatly increased through drinking alcohol or drug use[5].

HIV or AIDS does not afflict only gay[6] or bi-sexual[7] males. Today many women are becoming infected with AIDS, and, as a result, their babies are born HIV positive. Recently, there has been an increase in the number of heterosexual men and women who gotten HIV/AIDS. Many of these men and women got AIDS from having sex with more than one partner.

All citizens of the Navajo Nation must be educated about how to prevent HIV seropositivism or AIDS infection. Every person needs to know that AIDS is preventable. However, a promiscuous lifestyle and/or chemical dependency can place a person at a high risk of exposure to HIV or AIDS.

Traditional Navajo people have for years recognized that harmony with nature, community acceptance, group (extended family) support, and spirituality are essential to holistic healing practices. Disease prevention is a Navajo traditional concept; it is part of *hozhoji*[8], or unity and harmony. *'Adil 'idli*[8] (self

---

[5] Studies indicate that the consumption of alcohol and the use of drugs lowers a person's inhibitions and impair his/her reasoning. Persons under the influence of alcohol or drugs are more susceptible to avoiding safer sex precautions.

[6] "Gay" refers to homosexual men and women who are oriented to having sex with a partner or partners of the same sex.

[7] A "bisexual" is a person who has sexual relations with both men and women.

[8] Refer to Relevant Issues and Concerns, this Policy Statement, Page 11 and 12.

respect and value) *'adaa 'ati hat'ii*[10] (seeking holistic protection), and other traditional teachings are all a part of the concept. These traditional Navajo concepts are essential to the Policy Statement.

Navajo AIDS Policy Statement

The disease of AIDS shall be a top priority concern of all professionals responsible for addressing health, social, and related problems of the Navajo Nation. The medical costs for AIDS patient care are expensive. The Navajo Nation and the Navajo Area Indian Health Service (Indian Health Service) must make a strong commitment to secure funding to combat HIV and AIDS.

The Policy Statement is prevention-oriented and comprehensive in scope. It targets Navajo youth and others at risk. This Policy Statement is a Navajo Nation mandate to join other jurisdictions and the American health community to counsel, to educate, to provide compassionate medical treatment, and to protect individuals from discrimination or invasion of privacy. All Navajo Nation programs and services shall cooperate with the Policy Statement goals to prevent the spread of HIV/AIDS.

The Navajo Nation adopts the following policies and procedures related to HIV and AIDS issues:

---

[9] Id.

[10] Id.

1. <u>Equal Access to Services</u>

No person shall be denied services nor offered substandard services because of real or suspected HIV positive antibody status. There is no valid ethical, epidemiological, or legal reason for a program or business within the Navajo Nation to refuse service or to refuse to employ a person, testing HIV positive, who is otherwise qualified for service, benefit, or employment.

2. <u>HIV Education</u>

Education on AIDS prevention throughout the Navajo Nation is a top priority, along with efforts to combat the problem of alcoholism and substance abuse. A comprehensive AIDS education program, with resource materials will focus on behavioral change and shall be available to all citizens of the Navajo Nation. The purpose of AIDS education shall be to instill behavior which will help people from getting HIV or AIDS. AIDS education efforts shall prevent or eliminate personal fears and/or concerns about AIDS. The AIDS education program shall be undertaken by education, health social services and other programs to combat the spread of HIV and AIDS. Major HIV/AIDS education campaigns are to be planned and carried out on a regular basis by the Navajo Division of Health, the NAIHS, including other organizations, in various Navajo communities.

<u>- Navajo terminology in AIDS education</u>

Navajo terms to be used in AIDS education shall be as simple as possible. Instead of coining long Navajo terms to describe

"AIDS" or "HIV", AIDS education shall focus on getting the Navajo people used to the English acronyms "HIV" and "AIDS". Navajos have long adopted other acronyms, i.e., CCC, ONEO, CAC, and LCDP, so it should not be a problem to adopt two additional acronyms for AIDS education purposes.

However, the use of the terms "HIV" and "AIDS" does not prohibit use of the terms currently in use nor does it discourage refinement of better explanations of HIV and AIDS in the Navajo language.

- Education of Navajo leaders about AIDS

Currently, no Navajo law addressing HIV/AIDS exists. The Navajo Nation Council has not addressed HIV/AIDS as a social and medical issue.

All Navajo Nation Council delegates, chapter officers, and other elected officials of the Navajo Nation shall be educated on HIV and AIDS.

- Educators' role in AIDS education

Local school boards and parent advisory groups shall be educated to assist with AIDS prevention efforts in the schools. Lesson plans or curricula[11] shall be developed and implemented to allow for traditional Navajo values in AIDS education.

School boards without an AIDS policy shall require that AIDS education be structured with the curriculum at strategic grade levels. *'Adil 'idli* and other Navajo traditional teachings shall

[11] Similar to the "Navajo Beauty Way" and the Johns Hopkins University curriculum.

be incorporated in the education process wherever relevant. All school board policies on AIDS shall address the needs of students testing HIV positive and/or students already sick with HIV/AIDS. Parents, family members, and community leaders are to be involved in the education process as well.

3. Infection Control/Universal Precautions

It is unlikely a person can be at risk of HIV infection through occupational exposure to blood, semen, or vaginal secretions. All programs, services and businesses within the Navajo Nation, even if only for general hygienic reasons or to control infection by other blood-borne diseases, shall adopt simple, accessible infection control procedures, and establish a protocol within their organizations. The Navajo Occupational Safety and Health Administration, the Navajo Division of Health, and the NAIHS shall assist in the planning, implementation, maintenance, and monitoring of infection control procedures. These coordinated official programs shall be monitored to assure compliance with standards for continued operation.

4. HIV Antibody Testing

The Navajo Nation does not support mandatory HIV antibody testing. No person shall be forced to take an HIV antibody test. The Navajo Nation recognizes the many complicated issues related to mandatory HIV antibody testing, and leaves this decision to each individual. Service providers and others who have received appropriate HIV antibody test counseling training are responsible for assisting each person on the following:

a. To decide whether or not to be tested;

b. To educate each person in the language he or she understands about the reasons for HIV antibody testing and their respective advantages and disadvantages;

c. To provide adequate and appropriate follow-up counseling, or referral for counseling, before and after testing.

d. An explanation of the importance of partner notification.

Anonymous testing shall be made available within the Navajo Nation.

5. <u>Confidentiality and/or Anonymous Testing</u>[12]

A great deal of harm can be inflicted upon a person who tests HIV positive, or takes a test, and whose efforts or results are inappropriately or illegally disclosed to third parties[13]. In accordance with the Privacy Act of 1974 and the Americans with Disabilities Act of 1992, all programs, services, and businesses within the Navajo Nation shall insure the confidentiality of each person's HIV test status. All programs, services, and businesses within the Navajo Nation shall develop and adopt policies which address specific questions and issues concerning HIV antibody

---

[12] Arizona, New Mexico and Utah utilize "anonymous testing" for HIV determination which requires partner notification. The Indian Health Service utilizes a "confidentiality testing", which does not requires partner notification.

[13] Third parties are persons not officially involved in the treatment or counseling process.

status, including confidentiality. These policies shall address issues such as who needs to know when a client self-reports HIV seropositivity, program responsibilities and liabilities in relationship to HIV status information, third party disclosure, charting protocols of HIV status, and other matters.

6. There shall be Navajo Nation-wide coordination and networking of all AIDS combat efforts

The real success in addressing the problem of AIDS will come from everyone within the Navajo Nation. We must all work together for preserving the good health of future generations, and allow persons afflicted with AIDS to live their remaining years with respect and dignity. The Navajo Nation shall coordinate and direct all efforts to address the problems of HIV and AIDS infection in a comprehensive manner.

7. Policy Statement on NAIHS Medical Services for HIV-Positive Patients

HIV-positive patients require coordinated and complex medical care and social services. The Indian Health Service is the chief provider of direct medical services for the Navajo people. The Indian Health Service must be involved in the development of a comprehensive services for HIV-positive patients and their families.

Medical care and treatment provided by the Indian Health Service for HIV-positive patients shall be competent and compassionate. The Indian Health Service shall make special efforts to keep clinical services up-to-date with the recent developments in HIV/AIDS-related care. The Indian Health Service's medical care and treatment shall be compassion and respect the patient's wishes. Direct services will include, but not be limited to the following: HIV antibody testing and counseling; education about prevention of HIV-related complications, up-to date pharmacologic treatment for HIV infection and for the many other types of infection complicating HIV disease, mental health and counseling services for HIV, competent and compassionate medical care and treatment for both inpatients and outpatients, including their families, dental services, and assistance with navigating the medical systems of care when referral to tertiary care services is indicated by the patients medical condition and their wishes. The Indian Health Service will help to coordinate third-party resources and contact health services to make sure eligible patients can receive these services.

Health and social services providers of the Navajo Nation and the Indian Health Service shall be jointly responsible for developing a coordinated system of care for HIV-positive patients and their families. Local HIV-related resource listings shall be developed and made available to assist patients and non-medical providers in accessing the system of direct care services.

The Indian Health Service shall provide continuous quality improvement efforts to ensure that medical care and treatment is appropriate, respectful, and reflects current knowledge and clinical guidelines about HIV-related illness. A means for patient and family input into this Continuous Quality Improvement (CQI) program will be provided.

8. Additional resources shall be pursued

The Navajo Nation and the Indian Health Service shall seek additional resources necessary to address the problem of HIV/AIDS.

9. Amendments to the Policy Statement

The Navajo Nation, through the Navajo Division of Health, shall monitor the incidence of AIDS cases, identify alternative treatment programs and information about HIV and AIDS. The Navajo Division of Health will also inform all persons within the Navajo Nation of any changes to the Policy Statement. Any changes to this Policy Statement will be made, as necessary, to continue to address the devastating problem of AIDS. The Navajo Nation reserves the right to amend this Policy Statement pursuant to Title 2 of the Navajo Tribal Code.

Relevant Issues and Concerns

There is need to research old Navajo teachings and re-initiate the traditional ways of dealing with promiscuity, a major contributing factor in the spread of AIDS and other sexually transmitted diseases among teens and adults. Navajo traditional teachings may contribute in more ways to preventing the incidence of AIDS and other sexually transmitted diseases. These teachings may well be the sole means by which the Navajo Nation survives

AIDS. Western medicine has no cure for AIDS. Traditional Navajo healing may evolve as a primary means of treatment for persons already sick with AIDS. A key to this issue and concern is the position to be taken by the Dine' Spiritual Cultural Society, Inc.

Navajo Division of Health
OFFICE OF ENVIRONMENTAL HEALTH/CODE ENFORCEMENT

TESTIMONY

of

ENVIRONMENTAL HEALTH PROBLEM

Environmental Health Problems and Issues continue to be many and similar within communities and jurisdictions of local health department through out our country, however, within the Navajo Nation and other Indian Lands these problems and issues are by far greater. The primary responsibility and objective towards environmental health issues within Navajo Division of Health is to reduce the rates of morbidity and mortality from injuries and environmentally related diseases. Navajo Division of Health environmental health problems and issues encompass:

1. Injuries
2. Water and Sewer Service
3. Environmental Diseases
4. Solid Waste

INJURIES:

The leading cause of death among the Navajos is injuries. This is reflected in the statistical rate of the injuries occurring are at a rate 4.5 times the national average; a rate twice as high as the next leading cause—heart disease. The greatest numbers of injury death are seen from motor vehicles crashes. Falls, exposer, assaults, homicides, and suicides are other leading causes of injury. There have been joint measures initiated or conducted to address these problems, for example, successful programs to reduce motor vehicle injuries by increased seat belt use. In this same light, pedestrian fatalities have also been successfully reduces. From these efforts it has become even more evident that continued and committed efforts needs to be done to further effect reduction on motor vehicle injuries, assaults, homicides, suicides, spousal/child/elderly abuse, and exposure. Reported for 1993:

Accidents:	
With injuries	68
With deaths	49
Homicides:	15
Aggravated Assaults:	314
Assaults & Battery:	2,384
Sex Offenses:	364
Offenses/Family-Child:	576
Suicides & Attempts:	
first quarter-'94:	10
Suicides:	03
Attempts:	07

ENVIRONMENTAL DISEASES:

For the Navajo Nation and its people, environmental related diseases is a sincere and real concern. With the recent outbreak of hantavirus—a rodent-borne disease—it became evident that the cultural values of traditional environmental health in preventing disease must never be lost. Diseases of concerns include, but not limited to: Hepatitis A, Shigella, Salmonella, Plague, Rabies, and now Hantavirus. Congressional support in the form of adequate funding shall provide good sound environmental health programs to conduct effective practices. The provisions of potable water and waste disposal, proper sanitation procedures, food sanitation, monitoring environmental health conditions of schools, restaurants, hospitals, nursing homes, and water systems, surveillance of rodents carrying plague and hantavirus, and monitoring rabies all contribute to reducing rates of environmentally related diseases.

SOLID WASTE:

The Navajo Nation is not immune to the trails of visible blight that leaves few corners of our country unspotted of refuse on the land; litter along the roadside, abandoned vehicles, thousands of open dumps scarring the land. Residential, commercial, institutional, and industrial solid waste are the clearest threats to health and the environment, they are the most offensive and the most dangerous to health when allowed to accumulate near where people live. An overriding concern is the disposal of discarded hazardous waste—those which by virtue of their composition or longevity are harmful, toxic or lethal, therefore, presenting a clear danger to the health and safety of the population and to the quality of the environment.

On the Navajo Nation their are approximately 350 dump site that would qualify for the open dumps lists identifying priority sites for abatement measures. Of this number, 150 - 200 sites may be the subject of proper closure measures. The remaining would require corrective measures to upgrade and meet the required standards to remain operative. Not reflected herein are the thousands of small family camp site or community dumps, and illegal dumping areas. Congressional funding for clean-up, monitoring and surveillance, and enforcement are greatly needed. Progress to date; approximately 25 transfer stations have been established with approximately 10 additional transfer sites proposed for consideration in the near future. The approximate development cost per transfer site is $50,000.00. This cost does not include operating expenditure factors such as: Pick-up (pull cost) of dumpsters, transportation to and from sites (note, all sites most likely will be in a remote rural area), landfill disposal fees, site care and maintenance, and manpower at each site. In addition to the identified funding needed above, and for proper closure, corrective abatement measures, and continued operations there is needed funding for public education and enforcement programs. The priority of the Navajo Nation is to focus on the development of three (3) approved sanitary landfill sites. The approximate development cost is projected to be $3,000,000.00 (Three million) per landfill site; totalling $9,000,000.00 (Nine million).

The Navajo Nation through coordinated efforts of the Indian Health Services; CDC; Navajo OEH; NDOH CHR Program; Health Education; Special Projects NDOH; Division of Social Services and Health Departments from Arizona, New Mexico and Utah have continuously attempted to meet the health needs of the Navajo people, although the resources available continues to diminish due to a variety of reasons. In any case we as leaders have to continue advocating for those constituents.

CHILD ABUSE - GENEVIEVE JACKSON

The Navajo Child Sexual Abuse Project (NCSAP) is now in its third year of operation, but due to funding obstacles, the NCSAP has managed to implement only one full year of operation. Despite the late start intervention, prevention and culturally appropriate treatment services have been provided to 542 primary clientele (children). The U.S. Congress should join in these historic developments by appropriating monies for Public Law 101-630.

HANTA VIRUS ACTIVITIES - LYDIA HUBBARD-POURIER

This virus is probably as old as time, but there has been very little understanding of the epidemic that has occurred in and around Crownpoint; Shiprock; and basically the Four Corners Area, but the various component of the Health and Science communities have wrestled with this problem and are continuing since the onset of the crisis. There is discussion of conducting a research study with Ribavirin, because it is unknown whether this particular drug is effective enough to be authorized for use in the United States. The concept has been received with a lot of ethical questions, especially in consideration of the Navajo Traditions.

DEPARTMENT OF BEHAVIORAL HEALTH - NORMAN RATION

The Navajo DBHS provides and coordinates alcohol treatment programs through five agencies and several field offices in a geographic area of 27,000 square miles in size. Individual and group outpatient treatment and counseling services are provided to clients, youth and adults whose lives are affected by alcohol and substance abuse and associated problems. Mental health as an illness has been associated to alcoholism/substance abuse and requires appropriate facilitation as such to minimize its effects on the afflicted.

Various studies indicate that alcohol is a major contributing factor to morbidity and mortality in the leading disease categories of the Navajo people, but treatment programs which would address cultural sensitivity and holistic methods spiritually relevant to the Navajo client(s) is not readily available.

There are immediate needs for intense and structured facility services for chronic Navajo alcoholics who need the services of; short-term and long term rehabilitation, halfway houses and custodial care.

FACILITIES - PEGGY NAKAI

The Navajo Nation will continue to advocate and request Congressional appropriations to construct new health care facilities in the Navajo area. The Navajo Area IHS has the unique status of being one of the few remaining IHS areas across the country to continue to provide health care services to its Native American Indian population.

NAVAJO NATION AIDS OFFICE - ROSELYN CHAPELA

AIDS an incurable disease has adversely impacted the Native Americans, particularly women of child bearing age that is 4 to 8 times higher than of women in general population and recent reports indicate that there was 82 present increase in the number of persons tested for HIV between 1991 and 1992.

The Navajo Nation needs resources to continue to promote awareness and education to reduce and confine the spread of HIV

ENVIRONMENTAL HEALTH PROBLEMS - HERMAN SHORTY

The Navajo Nation has had open sanitary landfills, established by the Federal Agencies to accommodate solid waste (discarded materials) of major agency communities and rural areas from the increase of population. Solid waste, including liquid chemicals, threaten the underground aquifers. Residential, commercial, institutional, and industrial solid waste, though they make up a small part of the total load of solid waste generated, are the clearest threats to health and to the environment. They are the most offensive and the most dangerous to health when allowed to accumulate near where people live.

Salt River
PIMA-MARICOPA INDIAN COMMUNITY
ROUTE 1, BOX 216 / SCOTTSDALE, ARIZONA 85256-9722 / PHONE (602) 941-7277

February 15, 1994

The Honorable William Clinton
President of the United States
The White House
1600 Pennsylvania Avenue, NW
Washington, DC 20500

Dear President Clinton:

The Salt River Pima-Maricopa Indian Community (SRPMIC) is deeply concerned about recent decisions by the Clinton Administration to cut the staffing for the Indian Health Service (IHS). The SRPMIC is also concerned about the lack of coordination within the Clinton Administration between its efforts to include Indian tribes in the Health Security Act and its efforts to reduce the annual budget and staffing for the Indian Health Service.

The Salt River Pima-Maricopa Indian Community requests that you direct the Office of Management and Budget to issue a waiver under Executive Order 12839 so that IHS does not need to reduce its FTEs. Secretary Donna Shalala has requested a waiver from OMB on the IHS FTE reductions, but the OMB has requested a waiver from OMB on the Executive Order allows "exemptions necessary for the delivery of essential services and compliance with applicable law." Clearly, the Indian Health Service meets these criteria.

The Salt River Pima-Maricopa Indian Community also recommends that you appoint a staff person in the White House Office of Intergovernmental Affairs to address the contradictions between the Health Security Act (Title VIII, Subtitle D) and the reductions in the IHS budget and FTEs. The Health Security Act envisions a role for the IHS and tribal governments under the new health care system. The budget and FTE reductions being imposed on the IHS would make it impossible for tribes and the IHS to participate effectively in the Health Security Act.

The IHS, which delivers essential health services to Indian tribes, has been ordered to reduce its staffing by 1,099 FTEs by the end of 1995. The FTE reduction for the IHS would result in the loss of 7 percent of total IHS staff. The Public Health Service has ordered that IHS FTE reduction should minimize the impact on essential patient care. However, there is no way that the IHS can implement the FTE reduction without negatively impacting the delivery of quality health care in IHS and tribal inpatient and outpatient facilities.

The Department of Health and Human Services (DHHS) has been ordered to reduce total DHHS FTEs by 5,200 by the end of FY 1995, which is a reduction of 4 percent. The IHS has been ordered to reduce its staffing by 1,099 FTEs, which is a reduction of 7 percent. The IHS will end up absorbing 21 percent of the Department's total FTE reduction, which is inequitable.

The Salt River Pima-Maricopa Indian Community (SRPMIC) receives much of its outpatient and inpatient services from the Phoenix Indian Medical Center (PIMC). The PIMC is one of three regional referral centers in the IHS. The PIMC is a 147-bed facility which provides services to five tribes in Central Arizona. In addition, the PIMC provides referral and specialty services to 43 tribes in Arizona, Nevada and Utah with a service population of 106,663 Indian reservation residents.

The Congress has recognized that the PIMC is funded to meet only 60 percent of the health care need of the population it serves, according to a methodology established pursuant to the Indian Health Care Improvement Act. In the FY 1994 Interior Appropriations Act, the Congress provided additional funds to bring the PIMC up to 60 percent of needed funded. Given its large service population, its multifaceted role and its lack of resources, the staff of the PIMC are forced to maintain a heavy workload with seriously inadequate resources.

The FTE reduction plan of the IHS Phoenix Area calls for a reduction of 63 FTEs by the end of FY 1995. The housekeeping staff would be reduced by 31 FTEs. It is very difficult to operate the PIMC with its current workload. The PIMC facility was build to handle 40,000 outpatient visits per year, PIMC currently handles 161,043 outpatient visits per year. A reduction in the housekeeping staff would result in unsafe and unsanitary patient facilities.

The plan also calls for a reduction of 32 dietary positions. The Public Health Service has suggested that the IHS contract out the dietary functions. However, it is important for the Clinton Administration to understand that one important mission of the PIMC is to treat patients suffering from complications of diabetes. The dietary staff of the PIMC have a many years of training and experience in working with Indian patients and providing appropriate nutritional services in a manner which is compatible with the cultures and lifestyles of the

Indian patients. The loss of these trained and experienced staff would be a major setback for the treatment of diabetes among Central Arizona Tribes.

There appears to be a lack of coordination within the Clinton Administration regarding Federal policies for Indian health care. One on hand, the Clinton Administration's proposed Health Security Act envisions a role for the Indian Health Service and tribal governments in the national health care system that would be implemented in FY 1999 (Title VIII, Subtitle D). The Clinton Administration should be commended for working with Indian tribes on the provisions in the bill and for continuing its outreach efforts. However, if the IHS continues to be funded to meet only 75 percent of the need nationwide, then the IHS and tribal governments will be unable to provide the comprehensive benefits package. If the Clinton Administration continues to reduce the IHS budget and FTEs, then the IHS and tribal governments will be unable to participate in the Health Security Act. It appears that the "policy" side of the Clinton Administration is not coordinating with the "budget" side of the Administration, with respect to Indian health care.

We are counting on the Clinton Administration to maintain the Federal government's legal and moral commitment to improving health care for Indian tribes. Thank you for your attention to this very important matter.

Sincerely,

Ivan Makil

The Honorable Ivan Makil
President

cc: Mr. Ira Magaziner
Ms. Marcia Hale
Mr. David Kleinberg
Secretary Donna Shalala
Ms. Judith Feder
Dr. Philip Lee
Mr. Michael Lincoln
Arizona Congressional Delegation

YAVAPAI-APACHE TRIBE
P.O. BOX 1188 CAMP VERDE, ARIZONA 86322 PHONE (602) 567-3649

March 23, 1994

President William Clinton
The White House
1600 Pennsylvania Avenue, NW
Washington, DC 20500

Dear President Clinton,

Please find enclosed a copy of the resolution that was passed by the Yavapai-Apache Tribal Council on March 12, 1994. This resolution is regarding the funding and staffing reductions in the Indian Health Service.

This is extremely important to our Tribe. If this happens IHS will be reducing the programs that are available to us now. It seems that if this is taken away we are in a standstill for service for our Tribe. Our Tribe relies on Indian Health Service.

Please review this before this drastic change happens. Looking forward to a beneficial outcome.

Cordially,

YAVAPAI-APACHE TRIBE

Theodore Smith, Sr.
Tribal Chairman

c: Marcia Hale
Ira Magaziner
David Kleinberg
Honorable Donna Shalala
Judith Feder
Dr. Philip Lee
Michael Lincoln
Honorable Dennis DeConcini
Honorable John McCain
Honorable Sam Coppersmith
Honorable Ed Pastor
Honorable Bob Stump
Honorable Jon Kyl
Honorable Jim Kolbe
Honorable Karan English

RESOLUTION No. 23-94
OF THE GOVERNING BODY OF THE
YAVAPAI-APACHE NATION

FUNDING AND STAFFING REDUCTIONS IN THE INDIAN HEALTH SERVICE

WHEREAS, the Clinton Administration has ordered the Indian Health Service (IHS) to reduce its Full-Time Equivalent (FTE) staffing levels by 1,289 FTEs by 1995; and

WHEREAS, the IHS had 15,418 FTEs in FY 1993, which represented 11.9 percent of the 130,000 FTEs in the entire Department of Health and Human Services (DHHS); and

WHEREAS, the DHHS has been ordered to reduce total DHHS FTEs by 5,200 (-4 percent) by FY 1995, but the IHS has been ordered to reduce IHS staff by 1,099 FTEs (-9 percent), which is inequitable; and

WHEREAS, the IHS will end up absorbing one-fifth of the entire DHHS FTE reduction (1,009/5,200=21 percent), which is inequitable; and

WHEREAS, the Phoenix Area IHS has been ordered to reduce staffing in the Phoenix Area by 173 FTEs by the end of FY 1995; and

WHEREAS, the FTE reduction, if implemented in the Phoenix Area, will negatively impact the housekeeping and dietary services of 8 IHS hospitals which, in turn, will lower the quality of services available to Indian tribes in Arizona, Nevada and Utah; and

WHEREAS, the IHS FTE reductions will further reduce the resources for IHS programs which are funded at 75 percent of need; and

WHEREAS, President Clinton's proposed Health Security Act addresses the role of the IHS and tribal governments in the new national health care system while President Clinton's proposed budgets for the IHS will undermine the ability of the IHS and tribal governments to function in the new system; and

WHEREAS, there appears to be a lack of coordination between the Clinton Administration' Indian health care policies as reflected in the contradiction between the role envisioned for the IHS and tribal governments outlined in the Health Security Act and the proposed annual budgets for the IHS for fiscal years 1994 and 1995;

NOW THEREFORE BE IT RESOLVED, that the Inter Tribal Council of Arizona, the Inter Tribal Council of Nevada and the Tribal Governments in Utah, representing 43 tribal governments in the IHS Phoenix Area call upon President Clinton, the White House Office of Intergovernmental Affairs and the Office of Management and Budget to:

1. Grant a waiver to exempt the Indian Health Service from the FTE reductions under Executive Order 12839;

2. Stop the plans to reduce the IHS budget and FTEs during the next several years;

3. Appoint a full-time position in the White House Office of Intergovernmental Affairs to coordinate the Administration's policies on Indian health care, specifically the relationship between IHS/tribal participation in the Health Security Act and the annual budgets of the IHS for fiscal years 1995-1999;

4. Commit the Federal government to a four-year strategy to invest in Indian health care, with the goal of increasing the level of health care resources to 100 percent of need as defined in the Indian Health Care Improvement Act.

C E R T I F I C A T I O N

I hereby certified that the foregoing resolution was adopted by an affirmative vote of the Tribal Council, presented for approval on March 12, 1994, pursuant to the authority contained under the Constitution of the Yavapai-Apache Tribe, approved April 13, 1992.

Theodore Smith Sr

Theodore Smith, Sr., Chairman

ATTEST:

Karla Reimer

Karla Reimer, Tribal Secretary

THE
NAVAJO
NATION

P. O. DRAWER 308 • WINDOW ROCK, ARIZONA 86515 • (602) 871-6352-55

PETERSON ZAH
PRESIDENT

MARSHALL PLUMMER
VICE PRESIDENT

February 3, 1994

The Honorable Congressman Jon Kyl
UNITED STATES HOUSE OF REPRESENTATIVES
Washington, D.C. 20515

Dear Congressman Kyl:

I have been notified by the Navajo Area Indian Health Service (IHS) of President Clinton's call for reduction in the federal work force and severe budget cuts in the IHS. The Navajo Nation has supported the President's comprehensive health care plan to make health care available to all Americans. However, the proposed reductions are totally contrary to such a plan.

Preliminary indications from the provisional FTE ceiling numbers indicate the loss of up to 500 positions in the Navajo Area. I simply cannot find words to adequately describe the devastating effect this will have on my people. The Navajo Nation is not overserved. In fact, IHS nationally is funded at only 68% of the total health care need. Navajos have no alternative outpatient or inpatient resources available at which to seek health care. NO PRIVATE INSURANCE COMPANIES, PHYSICIANS, OR HEALTH CARE PROVIDERS SERVE THE RESERVATION COMMUNITIES AFFECTED BY THESE CUTBACKS. Presently, at IHS facilities, patient waiting lists are extensive. It is not uncommon for severely injured or ill patients to be transported on dirt roads up to a hundred miles to be seen at these facilities, which are now scheduled for huge reductions. If these reductions occur, the additional staff required for the new Shiprock Hospital, which has been so desperately needed, would be staffed at only 54%. There is simply no logic nor humanity in reducing health care services to those who so desperately need them, nor in expending millions of dollars to construct a needed hospital only to have it stand half vacant due to staff cuts.

In response to mounting pressures of the FTE cuts, budget limits and downsizing of government, IHS has begun its restructuring effort. Though we recognize a need for examination and restructuring of IHS, these proposed reductions of staff in the only health care system for Indian reservations mean that many Native American Health care professionals now serving their communities, will be put out of work. In the Navajo Nation, the numbers would be added to an unemployment rate of over 40% which ranges up to 10 times higher than the rest of America, depending on the season.

The Honorable Jon Kyl
February 3, 1994
Page Two

One of the "downsizing" options being aggressively considered under the IHS Restructuring Plan is the consolidation of the Navajo Area IHS office with the Albuquerque and the Phoenix IHS Area offices. This would put the agency out of touch with the very people it serves. At this time the Navajo IHS Area addresses the needs of the people and facilitates through frequent interaction with local Navajo health boards and communities.

The recent Hantavirus or "mystery illness" which recently devastated primarily Navajo citizens accentuates the need for increased, not decreased, dollars and staff to address our underserved population. Life expectancy among Navajos is well under the overall U.S. Life expectancy. Infant deaths of Navajos far exceed those of the overall U.S. population. It is predictable that if the IHS budget is reduced, as proposed, the resulting costs of the failure to address health needs in their early stages, and already at deficient levels, will result in an increase in serious illnesses and untold costs which eventually must be borne by the U.S. Federal government, the trustee of its Indian citizens.

When American Indians were driven off their lands and forced onto tiny reservations, they were assured through their Treaties, that they would be provided education and other services, including health care, in exchange for giving up their treasured lands. Now instead of continuing the progress begun over the last several years in delivering critical health care, the IHS has been directed, under the guise of FTE cuts, budget limits, and downsizing government to implement these astounding cuts with no appeal, no recourse and no alternative source of services.

In conclusion, my concern is that the U.S. government's promises to its American Indian citizens would be irreversibly breached if these cutbacks are allowed to occur. I assure you that other American Indian leaders will join me to advocate for the Federal government to meet its Federal obligation to deliver adequate and quality health care services to our Indian people.

I look forward to working with you to ensure the protection of health care of Americans Indians and Alaska Natives.

Sincerely,

THE NAVAJO NATION

Peterson Zah
President

The Legislative Branch
The Navajo Nation

Nelson Gorman, Jr.
Speaker of the
Navajo Nation Council

February 7, 1994

Honorable Senator Jon Kyl
2440 Rayburn House Office Building
Washington, D. C. 20515-0304

Dear Senator:

Greetings from Navajoland!

Enclosed please find a copy of Navajo Nation Council Resolution CJA-11-94.

The resolution opposes the Clinton Administration across-the-board staff reductions and requests the Federal Office of Management and Budget for a waiver for Navajo Area Indian Health Service based on the Navajo Nation's unique relationship with the United States Government, pursuant to the Treaty of 1868.

The Navajo Nation Council is extremely concerned about the proposed staff cuts as Indian Health Service is the main health care provider to one of the poorest and most at-risk populations in America, the American Indian/Alaska Natives, and the adverse effect this will have on quality patient care; therefore, it opposes any drastic staff reduction that would cause a decrease in service delivery to the Indian and the Navajo people.

The Navajo Nation Council seeks your assistance in opposing the Clinton Administration across-the-board staff reduction and requests that if a blanket waiver cannot be granted to the Navajo Area Indian Health Service, that the Clinton Administration exempt direct hands-on health care providers in its staff reduction plan.

Sincerely,

NAVAJO NATION COUNCIL

Genevieve Jackson

Genevieve Jackson, Chairperson
Health and Social Services Committee

Enclosure

CJA-11-94

Class "C" Resolution
No BIA Action Required.

RESOLUTION OF THE
NAVAJO NATION COUNCIL

Opposing the Clinton Administration Across-the-Board Staff Reductions and Requesting the Federal Office of Management and Budget for a Waiver for Navajo Area Indian Health Service

WHEREAS:

1. The Navajo Nation Council is the governing body of the Navajo Nation, pursuant to 2 N.T.C., Section 102 (a); and

2. The United States Government, through the Indian Health Service, is responsible for providing a comprehensive health services delivery system for the Navajo people, as provided for in the Navajo Nation Treaty of 1868; and

3. The Clinton Administration has determined to reduce the federal work force by 252,000 positions and has requested all federal agencies to make staff reductions to meet this goal over the next several years. The Navajo Nation is concerned that these staff reductions are not equitable; and

4. Rather than making reductions across the board, the Clinton Administration should consider waivers for direct health care programs such as the Indian Health Service, the National Institute of Health and Veteran and Military Health Facilities; and

5. The United States Department of Health and Human Services has targeted a maximum Full-Time Equivalent (FTE) staffing of 14,787 for FY 1994 for Indian Health Service. A request for a waiver and an FTE ceiling of 15,697 FTE's for Indian Health Service for Fiscal Year 1994 was denied; and

6. The Navajo Nation Council is extremely concerned about the proposed staff cuts as Indian Health Service is the main health care provider to one of the poorest and most at-risk populations in America, the American Indian/Alaska Natives, and the adverse effect this will have on quality patient care; therefore, it opposes any drastic staff reduction that would cause a decrease in service delivery to the Indian and the Navajo people; and

7. The Navajo Nation Council notes the irony of the proposed staff reductions; at the same time the Clinton Administration is proposing Health Care Reform which promises increased health care for Indian people who will be treated like all other American citizens. It is illogical to strip the Indian Health Service health care system while also planning to increase health services to all Americans and Indian people within one or two years; and

8. It is very evident to local Navajo tribal leaders and consumers that large staff reductions will negatively affect health care delivery. Drastic staff cuts will cause longer waiting times, postponement or denial of needed medical care, decreased continuity of care and quality of care, greater staff turnover of medical staff who do not have adequate backup and service unit administrative support; and

9. In addition, large staff reductions will further exacerbate the lack of employment on the Navajo Nation affecting families who depend on said employment; further, Navajo education dollars spent for educating our youth in medical professions will not provide benefits here on the Navajo Nation; and

10. The Health and Social Services Committee of the Navajo Nation Council, by Resolution HSSC-JA-04-94, attached hereto as Exhibit "A", recommends opposition of the Clinton Plan for staff reduction.

NOW THEREFORE BE IT RESOLVED THAT:

1. The Navajo Nation Council hereby opposes the Clinton Administration across-the-board staff reduction and requests the Federal Office of Management and Budget to reconsider the waiver for the Navajo Area Indian Health Service based on the Navajo Nation's unique relationship with the United States Government, pursuant to the Treaty of 1868.

2. The Navajo Nation Council requests that if a blanket waiver cannot be granted to the Navajo Area Indian Health Service, that the Clinton Administration exempt direct "hands-on" health care providers in its staff reduction plan. There is currently an FTE ceiling on GS 14/15's and 0-6 commissioned officers. These positions and grades are necessary to attract doctors and specialized health professionals to the Navajo Area Indian Health Service.

3. The Navajo Nation Council also solicits support of this Navajo Nation waiver request from all federal programs, agencies and all appropriate committees of Congress, as well as each state Congressional delegation.

CERTIFICATION

I hereby certify that the foregoing resolution was duly considered by the Navajo Nation Council at a duly called meeting at Window Rock, Navajo Nation (Arizona), at which a quorum was present and that same was passed by a vote of 67 in favor, 1 opposed and 0 abstained, this 21st day of January 1994.

Nelson Gorman, Jr., Speaker
Navajo Nation Council
January 26, 1994
Date Signed

Motion: Sampson Begay
Second: Wallace Tsosie

ACTION BY THE EXECUTIVE BRANCH

1. Pursuant to 2 N.T.C. Section 1005 (c)(1), I hereby sign into law the foregoing legislation on this 27 day of January 1994:

Peterson Zah, President
Navajo Nation

* * * *

2. Pursuant to 2 N.T.C. Section 1005 (c)(10), I hereby veto the foregoing legislation this ____ day of __________ 1994 for the reason(s) expressed in the attached letter to the Speaker:

Peterson Zah, President
Navajo Nation

Health Care Reform which promises increased health care for Indian people who will be treated like all other American citizens. It is illogical to essentially strip the Indian Health Service health care system while planning to increase health services to all Americans and Indian people within one or two years; and

8. It is very evident to local Navajo tribal leaders and consumers that large staff reductions will negatively affect Health Care Delivery. Drastic staff cuts will cause longer waiting times; postponement or denial of needed medical care, decreased continuity of care and quality of care, greater staff turnover of medical staff who do not have adequate backup and service unit administrative support.

NOW THEREFORE BE IT RESOLVED THAT:

1. The Health and Social Services Committee of the Navajo Nation Council recommends to the Navajo Nation Council strong opposition to the Clinton Administration's across-the-board staff reductions and to request a waiver for the Indian Health Service.

2. The Health and Social Services Committee of the Navajo Nation Council further recommends that if the Clinton Administration must implement a federal employee reduction plan based on concerns of administrative costs, then they should target administrative staff and exempt direct "hands on" health care providers. There is currently an FTE ceiling on GS 14/15s and 0-6 commissioned officers. These positions and grades are necessary to attract doctors and specialized health professionals.

CERTIFICATION

I hereby certify that the foregoing resolution was duly considered by the Health and Social Services Committee of the Navajo Nation Council at a duly called meeting at Window Rock, Navajo Nation, Arizona, at which a quorum was present and that same was passed by a vote of 7 in favor, 0 opposed and 0 abstentions on this 20th day of January 1994.

Genevieve Jackson

Chairperson
Health and Social Services Committee
NAVAJO NATION COUNCIL

MOTION: Annie Descheny
SECOND: Harry Hubbard

78-786 - 94 - 10

HSSC-JA-04-94

RESOLUTION OF THE
HEALTH AND SOCIAL SERVICES COMMITTEE OF THE
NAVAJO NATION COUNCIL

Recommending to the Navajo Nation Council to Oppose the Clinton Administration Across-the-Board Staff Reductions and Requesting a Waiver for Indian Health Service

WHEREAS;

1. Pursuant to 2 N.T.C. Sections 451 and 454 (b) (1), the Health and Social Services Committee is hereby established as a standing committee of the Navajo Nation Council empowered to represent the Navajo Nation in matters relating to health, social services and environmental health; and

2. Pursuant to 2 N.T.C. Section 454 (b) (3), the Health and Social Services Committee is empowered to coordinate all health and social services related activities of the Navajo Nation and its enterprises, relating to delivery of health and social services and health and social services planning and prevention; and

3. The Clinton Administration has determined to reduce the federal workforce by 252,000 positions and has requested all federal agencies to make staff reductions to meet this goal over the next several years. While the Navajo Nation supports the goal of the President to reduce the cost of federal government, the Navajo Nation is concerned that these staff reductions are not equitable; and

4. Rather than making reductions across the board, the Administration should consider waivers for direct health care programs such as the Indian Health Service, the National Institute of Health, and the Veteran and Military Health Facilities; and

5. The United States Department of Health and Human Services has targeted a maximum Full-Time Equivalent (FTE) staffing of 14,787 positions for Indian Health Service for Fiscal Year 1994. A request for a waiver and an FTE ceiling of 15,697 FTEs for Indian Health Service for Fiscal Year 1994 was denied; and

6. The Health and Social Services Committee of the Navajo Nation Council is deeply concerned with these proposed staff cuts and the adverse affect this will have on quality patient care and opposes any drastic staff reduction that would cause a decrease in service delivery to the Indian and the Navajo people; and

7. The Health and Social Services Committee of the Navajo Nation Council notes the irony of the proposed staff reductions while at the same time the Clinton Administration is proposing

The Legislative Branch
The Navajo Nation

Nelson Gorman, Jr.
Speaker of the
Navajo Nation Council

March 3, 1994

The Honorable Representative Jon Kyle
2440 Rayburn House Office Building
Washington, D.C. 20515-0304

Dear Honorable Representative:

Enclosed please find the following resolutions of the Ooljee 'To Chapter and Sheep Spring Chapter of the Navajo Nation:

1. Ooljee 'To and Sheep Spring Chapters: Adopting and Approving the Opposition of Cuts in the Indian Health Service Staffing and Programs on the Navajo Nation and Indian Country.

2. Sheep Spring Chapter: Requesting the Indian Health Service to Include Funds in its Budget of $23,610,175 for Additional 515 Positions for the Northern Navajo Medical Center, Shiprock, New Mexico and

   Requesting the United States Congress to Include in the Fiscal Year 1995 Federal Budget Add-on Funds of $23,610,175 for Additional 515 Positions for the Northern Navajo Medical Center, Shiprock, New Mexico.

The Navajo Nation is extremely concerned about the proposed budget cuts within the Indian Health Service and non-funding of additional positions needed at the Northern Navajo Medical Center. Thus, the enclosed resolutions request your assistance in opposing the budget cuts in the Indian Health Service staffing and programs within the Navajo Nation, and obtaining funding for the additional positions required to provide comprehensive health care services at the Northern Navajo Medical Center.

Sincerely,

NAVAJO NATION COUNCIL

Genevieve Jackson

Genevieve Jackson, Chairperson
Health and Social Services Committee

Enclosures

OL02-050-94

Ooljee 'To Chapter
THE DINE' NATION

RECEIVED
[illegible]
CHAPTER GOVERNMENT
NATION BLDG. PROGRAM

Walter D. Atene, Council Delegate
Jackson Gillis, President
Henry Phillips, Vice President
James Adakai, Secretary / Treasurer
Herman Daniels, Grazing Committee

RESOLUTION OF THE OLJATO CHAPTER

Adopting and Approving the Opposition of Cuts in the Indian Health Service Staffing and Programs on the Navajo Nation and Indian Country.

WHEREAS, The Oljato Chapter, under the authority of the Navajo Nation Tribal Council, is a sovereign and recognized Chapter entity under the Navajo Nation Tribal Government, whose primary purpose is to protect the health, safety and welfare of the Navajo people within it's jurisdiction; and,

WHEREAS, Policy direction and administrative decisions regarding restructuring of the Federal Government by President Clinton's administration has created uncertainty and instability in the direct health care services to the Navajo people and other Indian Tribes; and,

WHEREAS, The Oljato Chapter is a strong advocate of the following:
- a) Indian Health Care is a treaty obligation of the United States Government.
- b) Indian Health Service is the designated primary Health Care provider of the Navajo people and other Indian Tribes.
- c) Health Care should not be diminished, for sovereign tribal entities and native communities, due to stipulations under the umbrella of treaty obligations; and,

WHEREAS, The Oljato Chapter is in [illegible] to the following:
- a) Any cuts in the 1994-95 budget affecting the delivery of health care to the Navajo people.
- b) The projected 1994-95 reduction in staffing of Indian Health Service on administration and direct service personnel that adversely affects the health care of the Navajo people.
- c) Relocation of the Navajo Area Indian Health Service away from the Navajo Nation property.
- [illegible] planning or actions regarding restructuring [illegible] the [illegible] Administration [illegible] Indian Health Service [illegible] consultation [illegible] the Navajo Nation and other Indian [illegible]

NOW THEREFORE BE IT RESOLVED [illegible] the Oljato Chapter recommends that the Navajo Nation Council take the following actions to insure the Clinton Administration protects the health and welfare of the Navajo people and other Indian Tribe by supporting [illegible] Health Service:

- a) Waive/exempt all planned [illegible]
- b) Waive/exempt all planned budget cuts.
- c) Equity and parity funding for Indian Health Service to the level of non-Indian health care facilities.
- d) Funding level at $6.335 billion over the next five years to allow

P. O. BOX 360455 - PH: (801) 727-3259 - FAX: (801) 727-3380 - MONUMENT VALLEY, UTAH 84536

Indian Health Service to provide comprehensive health benefits.

e) Meeting be held with the President and his key management staff on Health Care to include:
   1. First Lady Hillary Rodhan Clinton
   2. Donna Shalala
   3. Philip Lee
   4. Leon Panetta
   5. John Hart
   6. Loretta Avante
   7. Grag Stepanoupoulus

f) Meetings with Senate and Congressional committees having jurisdiction over Indian Health Care.

BE IT FURTHER RESOLVED that Oljato Chapter recommends the Navajo Nation and other Indian Tribes direct President Clinton and the U.S. Government to adhere to the Federal Indian Policy of continuous tribal consultation with elected tribal officials and Tribal sovereign governments in decisions regarding Indian policy and the affects on Indian people. That the Indian Health Service be allowed to improve the delivery of quality health care to it's Native American clients without fear of budget cuts and staff reduction.

C E R T I F I C A T I O N

We hereby certify that the foregoing resolution was duly considered by the Oljato Chapter at a duly called meeting in Oljato, Navajo Nation, Utah, at which a quorum was present and that same was passed by a vote of 59 in favor, and Ø opposed, that 13 day of February 1994.

Jackson Gillis
Jackson Gillis, President

Henry Phillips, Sr., Vice-President

James Adakai
James Adakai, Sec/Treasurer

Walter D. Atene
Walter D. Atene, Council Delegate

FYI

Chief Executive Officer
SRSU/Shiprock Hospital

Sheep Springs Chapter

P.O. Drawer "I" • Sheep Springs, NM 87364 • District 12
(505) 732-4288

RESOLUTION

ADOPTING AND APPROVING THE OPPOSITION OF CUTS IN THE INDIAN HEALTH SERVICE STAFFING AND PROGRAMS ON THE NAVAJO NATION AND INDIAN COUNTRY

WHEREAS:

1. The Sheep Springs Chapter, under the authority of the Navajo Nation Tribal Council, is a sovereign and recognized Chapter entity under the Navajo Nation Tribal Government, whose primary purpose is to protect the health, safety and welfare of the Navajo people within it's jurisdiction; and,

2. Policy direction and administrative decisions regarding restructuring of the Federal Government by President Clinton's administration has created uncertainty and instability in the direct health care services to the Navajo people and other Indian Tribes; and,

3. The Sheep Springs Chapter is a strong advocate of the following:
   a) Indian Health Care is a treaty obligation of the United States Government.
   b) Indian Health Service is the designated primary health Care provider of the Navajo people and other Indian Tribes.
   c) Health Care should not be diminished, for sovereign tribal entities and native communities, due to stipulations under the umbrella of treaty obligations; and

4. The Sheep Springs Chapter is in total opposition to the following:
   a) Any cuts in the 1994-5 budget affecting the delivery of health care to the Navajo people.
   b) The projected 1994-5 reduction in staffing of Indian Health Service in administration and direct service personnel that adversely affects the health care of the Navajo people.
   c) Relocation of the Navajo Area Indian Health Service away from the Navajo Nation property.
   d) Any further planning or actions regarding restructuring by the Clinton Administration regarding Indian Health Service without consultation with the Navajo Nation and other Indian Tribes.

NOW THEREFORE BE IT RESOLVED:

1. The Sheep Springs Chapter recommends that the Navajo Nation Council take the following actions to insure the Clinton Administration protects the health and welfare of the Navajo people and the Indian Tribes by supporting the Indian Health Service:

   a) Waive/exempt all planned staffing cuts.
   b) Waive/exempt all planned budget cuts.
   c) Equity and parity funding of Indian Health Service to the level of non-Indian health care facilities.

d) Funding level at $6.335 billion over the next five years to allow Indian Health Service to provide comprehensive health benefits.

e) Meeting be held with the President and his key management staff on Health Care to include:
   1. First Lady Hillary Rodham Clinton
   2. Donna Shalala
   3. Philip Lee
   4. Leon Panetta
   5. John Hart
   6. Loretta Avante
   7. Greg Stepanoupoulus

f) Meetings with Senate and Congressional committees having jurisdiction over Indian Health Care.

2. The Sheep Springs Chapter recommends the Navajo Nation and other Indian Tribes direct President Clinton and the U.S. Government to adhere to the Federal Indian Policy of continous tribal consultation with elected tribal officials and Tribal sovereign governments in decisions regarding Indian policy and the affects on Indian people. That the Indian Health Service be allowed to improve the delivery of quality health care to its Native American clients without fear of budget cuts and staff reduction.

CERTIFICATION

We, hereby, certify that the foregoing resolution was dicussed, considered and thus supported by Sheep Springs Chapter at a duly called meeting at Sheep Springs, Navajo Nation, New Mexico, at which a quorum was present and that same was passed by a vote of 31 in favor, and 0 opposed, on this 13th day of February 94.

Leonard H. Sandman
Leonard H. Sandman, President

Kenneth Denetclaw Sr.
Kennth Denetclaw Sr., Vice-President

Edison Wood
Edison Woods, Sec/Treas.

John A. Gould Sr.
John A. Gould Sr., Council Delegate

FYI
Chief Executive Officer
SRSU/Shiprock Hospital

Resolution of the ____Sheep Springs____ Chapter

REQUESTING THE INDIAN HEALTH SERVICES TO INCLUDE FUNDS INTO ITS BUDGET OF $23,610,175 FOR ADDITIONAL 515 POSITIONS FOR THE NORTHERN NAVAJO MEDICAL CENTER, SHIPROCK, NEW MEXICO

REQUESTING THE U.S. CONGRESS TO INCLUDE INTO THE FISCAL YEAR 1995 FEDERAL BUDGET ADD-ON FUNDS OF $23,610,175 FOR ADDITIONAL 515 POSITIONS FOR THE NORTHERN NAVAJO MEDICAL CENTER, SHIPROCK, NEW MEXICO

WHEREAS:

1. Pursuant to Resolution ________ of the Navajo Tribal Council, the ____Sheep Springs____ Chapter has been certified as a recognized body of the Navajo Nation and authorized to conduct business of the local government; and

2. The replacement of the Shiprock Indian Hospital has been in the plans for many years. The project finally commenced in 1987 when Congress appropriated the design funds. Construction funds was appropriated subsequently and construction will be completed on August 1, 1994; and

3. Using the upgraded Indian Health Services Staffing Methodology, the Navajo Area Indian Health Services requested 515 positions in December 1993 for the new Northern Navajo Medical Center. However, the President's Budget for Fiscal Year 1995 does not show any new positions for the Northern Navajo Medical Center; and

4. No new positions for the Northern Navajo Medical Center would have a devastating effect on the health care delivery system for the Navajo Indians. Examples, longer waiting time, exceeding 3 to 4 hours; no doctors and nurses will compound the existing manpower shortage; our immunization level falling below 95%; our infant mortality rate dropping below the national average; termination of several inpatient services and public health services; sending our people off the reservation to hospitals that are not culturally sensitive, nor speak the language of our people; cessation of the much needed health promotion and disease prevention activities, etc; and

5. A majority of our people have to travel more than 2 hours on dirt roads to access any medical care on the Navajo reservation. The new Northern Navajo Medical Center is the only Indian Health Hospital available to the Indian people of Northern Navajo.

NOW, THEREFORE BE IT RESOLVED THAT:

1. The Sheep Springs Chapter hereby request the Indian Health Services to include funds into its budget of $23,610,175 for additional 515 positions for the Northern Navajo Medical Center, Shiprock, New Mexico.

2. The Sheep Springs Chapter hereby request of the U.S. Congress to include into the Fiscal Year 1995 Federal Budget add-on funds of $23,610,175 for additional 515 positions for the Northern Navajo Medical Center, Shiprock, New Mexico.

CERTIFICATION

We, hereby certify that the foregoing resolution was duly considered by the Sheep Springs Chapter at a duly called meeting at ~~Shiprock,~~ New Mexico, at which a quorum was present and that the same was passed by a vote of 31 in favor and 0 opposed, and 6 abstained, this 13th of February '94 1994.

Leonard Sandoman
President

Council Delegate

Kenneth Benaldaw Sr.
Vice President

Council Delegate

Edison Wood
Secretary

[signature]
Council Delegate

IMPACT STATEMENT

NO NEW POSITIONS FOR THE NEW NORTHERN NAVAJO MEDICAL CENTER

Using the upgraded Indian Health Service Staffing Methodology, the Navajo Area Indian Health Service requested 515 positions in December 1993 for the new Northern Navajo Medical Center. However, President Clinton's Budget for Fiscal Year 1995 does not show any new positions for the Northern Navajo Medical Center.

No new positions for the Northern Navajo Medical Center would have a devastating effect on the health care delivery system for the Navajo Indians. The following are examples of what it would mean to our people if we do not get additional staffing for our new hospital:

1. A majority of our people have to travel more than two hours on dirt roads to access medical care on the Navajo Reservation. If the Northern Navajo Medical Center is not staffed with health care professionals, where would we go for medical treatment and care that is equivalent to President Clinton's Universal Benefits Package for United States citizens?

2. Another broken promise by our United States Government, our new hospital will simply become a newer, bigger place where nothing has really changed. We will still have to wait even longer hours to see a doctor and will not be able to see the same doctor as there will be no new doctors and nurses for the new hospital.

3. There will be no ear, nose and throat (ENT) surgery. Currently, there are only two ENT physicians for the Navajo area. Our young patients who need "ear tubes" for recurrent ear infections, older patients with ruptured eardrums who need repair, and others needing ENT speciality services would benefit greatly from our own ENT physician. We currently have an ENT doctor interested in working at the new hospital who is also trained in plastic surgery. His skills would be an immense benefit to our many patients with burns and injuries who need reparative services. ENT specialists are in high demand and, if we do not hire this physician, we may not be able to recruit one soon because doctors are exxremely difficult to recruit to the Indian Health Service.

4. There will be no on-site orthopedic surgery. Our greatest need is operative repair of traumatic bone injuries, as well as, non-operative follow-up of these injuries. The high rate of intentional and unintentional injuries among our people has been well documented. Currently, the Gallup Indian Medical Center provides follow-up clinical services once a month to a large number of patients. There are no operative orthopedics services on site.

5. Expanded scope and volume of dental services and optometry services to meet increasing needs of our growing population are planned for at the new hospital. Without dental and optometry staff, we will have to limit such services even more as our population expands. Already we have our people lined up for hours to obtain dental or optometry appointments. Currently, we are not able to provide prosthodontics services. We only provide to a limited portion of the population ongoing "routine" dental care. We will become more and more an "emergencies only" dental and optometry clinics. There is no system available for contracting dentistry and optometry services as we do not have an option to do so.

6. Most critical, without additional doctors and nursing staff in the outpatient department, we will not be able to offer our patients the improvements in continuity of care that have been planned for the new hospital. The majority of our 140,000 outpatient visits currently are non-appointed visits, they are walk-ins, through the treatment room. For our people, this means longer waiting times in an overcrowded waiting area; seeing different doctors every time; talking about sensitive personal issues in a busy room sectioned off by a curtain; and little time for attention to routine or preventive care. In planning the new hospital, we listened carefully to our people's concerns, complaints and suggestions and designed a system wherein most patients would be seen by their doctors. We will not be able to make these improvements to the high volume service delivery (outpatient care) if we do not have additional nurses and nursing assistants to make it work. Without additional staff, the United States Government is setting itself for failure to provide adequate, safe, and respectful health care services to Native Americans.

7. Without additional administrative-support staff, we have to limit clinical services to even less than what we have now. Do we now ask our doctors, nurses and other direct care providers to do their own clerical work, expedite their own travel orders, process their own payroll, order their own supplies, procure their own patient supplies, clean patient, examination and operating rooms?

8. We planned for the construction of an audiology clinic in the new hospital; however, without staff to man the clinic, there will be no services provided to the people.

9. After much hard work justifying the need, we are installing a CT scanner in the new hospital. Currently, many of our patients have to travel many miles for CT scans. Without additional staff in radiology, we will be unable to use the new scanner or cut back on other services within the radiology department to staff the scanner. By doing so, the patients are further inconvenienced and some very sick patients will be required to take the risks of traveling long distances for services. The new hospital will have the necessary equipment and facility to provide this service; however, staffing is required.

10. Currently, we have begun to emphasize prevention, both in the clinic and the community. With limited resources and staffing, this will become even more important. Our efforts have focused on adolescent health, school health education, women's health, injury prevention, AIDS prevention, nutrition and exercise, and domestic violence prevention. There will be pressure to cut back on prevention and health promotion efforts as health resources become limited and services are confined to emergency medical care only. Terminating or decreasing health prevention and health promotion efforts will be a great loss to our communities as well as to the patients we serve. We believe that prevention is an effective tool in addressing the growing health and social problems, i.e. violent deaths and injuries, child and partner abuse, increasing cases of diabetes-related amputations, increasing cases of kidney and heart diseases, etc. As we are just beginning to see diabetes among our children, we have re-dedicated ourselves to prevention. Without new staff, we risk losing this commitment and vision to building a healthier Navajo Nation.

11. Last, but not least, the United States Government is once again reneging on a solemn promise and agreement with sovereign nations. Legal binding agreements were entered into in good faith between our forefathers and the United States Government; hence, the justification for the sole existence of the Indian Health Service and the Northern Navajo Medical Center should not be based on need, poverty, or remoteness, but on a promise. Despite this, there is a great health care need and **no real alternative** available to meet the need.

19 TRIBES

INTER TRIBAL COUNCIL of ARIZONA, INC.

MEMBER TRIBES
AK-CHIN COMMUNITY
CAMP VERDE YAVAPAI APACHE INDIAN COMMUNITY
COCOPAH TRIBE
COLORADO RIVER INDIAN TRIBES
FORT McDOWELL YAVAPAI TRIBE
FORT MOJAVE TRIBE
GILA RIVER INDIAN COMMUNITY
HAVASUPAI TRIBE
HOPI TRIBE
HUALAPAI TRIBE
KAIBAB-PAIUTE TRIBE
TOHONO O'ODHAM NATION
PASCUA YAQUI TRIBE
QUECHAN TRIBE
SALT RIVER PIMA MARICOPA INDIAN COMMUNITY
SAN CARLOS APACHE TRIBE
TONTO APACHE TRIBE
WHITE MOUNTAIN APACHE TRIBE
YAVAPAI PRESCOTT INDIAN TRIBE

February 11, 1994

The Honorable Jon Kyl
US House of Representatives
2440 Rayburn House Building
Washington, DC 20515

Dear Representative Kyl,

Enclosed is a copy of a letter that the Inter Tribal Council of Arizona (ITCA) has sent to President Clinton regarding the impacts of the FTE reductions on the Indian Health Service. The ITCA has asked President Clinton to direct the Office of Management and Budget (OMB) to approve a waiver for IHS from the FTE reductions.

The Clinton Administration has ordered the IHS to reduce its total staffing by 1,099 FTEs (-7%) by the end of FY 1995. The Department of Health and Human Services has been ordered to reduce total DHHS FTEs by 5,200 FTEs (-4%). If the plan is implemented, the IHS will absorb one-fifth of the entire Department's FTE reduction.

The Phoenix Area IHS has been ordered to cut 193 FTEs. There is no way that the Phoenix Area can cut 193 FTEs without negative impacts on the Phoenix Indian Medical Center, 7 other hospitals and 15 clinics in Arizona, Nevada and Utah.

Thank you for your assistance in this matter.

Sincerely,

Dale Phillips

Dale Phillips
President, The Inter Tribal Council of Arizona
Chairman, The Cocopah Tribe

4205 North 7th Avenue · Suite 200 · Phoenix, Arizona 85013 · (602) 248-0071 Fax (602) 248-0080

19
TRIBES

INTER TRIBAL COUNCIL of ARIZONA, INC.

February 10, 1994

The Honorable William Clinton
President of the United States
The White House
1600 Pennsylvania Avenue, NW
Washington, DC 20500

Dear President Clinton,

The Inter Tribal Council of Arizona, Inc. is concerned about decisions by the Administration to cut the staffing for the Indian Health Service (IHS). The Inter Tribal Council of Arizona, Inc. (ITCA) is also concerned about the lack of coordination within the Clinton Administration regarding Federal policies for Indian health care.

The ITCA requests that you direct the Office of Management and Budget to approve a waiver under Executive Order 12839 to exempt the IHS from the FTE reductions. Secretary Donna Shalala has requested a waiver on the IHS FTE reductions, but the OMB has denied the waiver. The Executive Order allows "exemptions necessary for the delivery of essential services and compliance with applicable law." Clearly, the Indian Health Service meets these criteria.

The ITCA also recommends that you appoint a staff person in the White House Office of Intergovernmental Affairs to coordinate the Administration's Indian health care policies. On one hand, the Clinton Administration has made positive efforts to work with Indian tribes and to include provisions in the Health Security Act (Title VIII, Subtitle D) for IHS and tribal participation under the national health care system. On the other hand, the reductions in the IHS budget and FTEs proposed by the Clinton Administration will undermine the ability of the IHS and tribal governments to participate effectively in the Health Security Act.

The IHS has been ordered to reduce its staffing by 1,099 FTEs by the end of FY 1995. The FTE reduction for the IHS would result in a loss of 7 percent of total IHS staff.

4205 North 7th Avenue · Suite 200 · Phoenix, Arizona 85013 · (602) 248-0071 Fax (602) 248-0080

The Department of Health and Human Services (DHHS) has been ordered to reduce total DHHS FTEs by 5,200 by the end of FY 1995, which is a reduction of 4 percent. Because the IHS must reduce its FTEs by 1,099, the IHS will end up absorbing one-fifth of the Department's total FTE reduction, which is inequitable.

The Phoenix Area Indian Health Service includes 41 tribal governments with lands located in Arizona, Nevada and Utah. There are 10 Service Units in the Phoenix Area. The IHS operates 7 inpatient hospitals in the Phoenix Area.

In addition, the IHS operates the Phoenix Indian Medical Center (PIMC), which is a 147-bed facility which provides referral and specialty services to 41 tribes in Arizona, Nevada and Utah with a service population of 106,663 Indian reservation residents.

The Congress has recognized that the PIMC is funded to meet only 60 percent of the health care need of the population it serves, according to a methodology established pursuant to the Indian Health Care Improvement Act. In the FY 1994 Interior Appropriations Act, the Congress provided additional funds to bring the PIMC up to 60 percent of need funded. Given its large service population, its complex responsibilities and its lack of resources, the staff of the PIMC are forced to maintain a heavy workload with seriously inadequate resources.

The IHS FTE reduction plan calls for a reduction of 63 FTEs at the PIMC by the end of FY 1995. The housekeeping staff would be reduced by 31 FTEs. It is very difficult to operate the PIMC with its current workload. The PIMC facility was build to handle 40,000 outpatient visits per year; PIMC currently handles 160,000 outpatient visits per year. A reduction in the housekeeping staff would result in unsafe and unsanitary patient care facilities.

The plan also calls for a reduction of 32 dietary positions. The Public Health Service has suggested that the IHS contract out the dietary functions. However, it is important for the Clinton Administration to understand that one important mission of the PIMC is to treat patients suffering from complications of diabetes. The dietary staff of the PIMC have many years of experience in working with Indian patients and providing nutritional services and counseling in a manner which is compatible with the cultures and lifestyles of the Indian patients. The loss of 32 trained and experienced staff would be a major setback for the treatment of diabetes among Central Arizona tribes.

The IHS also operates, either directly, or through Self-Determination contracts with tribal governments, 15 health clinics and health stations in the Phoenix Area. In Nevada, the IHS FTE reduction plan calls for the elimination of the pharmacy staff, which supports the operation of several tribal health clinics. If the tribal health clinics are forced to contract individually with private providers in Nevada, the costs for prescription drugs will increase dramatically and Indian people will experience difficulties filling their prescriptions especially in remote Nevada Indian communities.

The IHS Phoenix Area has been ordered to reduce its FTEs by 193 by the end of FY 1995. The Public Health Service has ordered that the IHS FTE reduction should minimize the impact on essential patient care. However, there is no way that the IHS can implement the FTE reduction without negatively impacting the delivery of quality health care in IHS and tribal inpatient and outpatient facilities.

There appears to be a lack of coordination within the Clinton Administration regarding Federal policies for Indian health care. The Clinton Administration's health care task force worked with Indian people to develop provisions in the Health Security Act that would provide a role for the Indian Health Service and tribal governments in the national health care system that would be implemented in FY 1999 (Title VIII, Subtitle D). However, if the IHS continues to be funded to meet only 75 percent of Indian health care needs, then the IHS and tribal governments will be unable to provide the comprehensive benefits package proposed in the Health Security Act.

We are counting on the Clinton Administration to maintain the Federal government's legal and moral commitment to improve health care for Indian tribes. Thank you for your attention to this very important matter.

Sincerely,

Dale Phillips

The Honorable Dale Phillips
President, The Inter Tribal Council of Arizona
Chairman, The Cocopah Tribe

cc: Mr. Ira Magaziner
Ms. Marcia Hale
Mr. David Kleinberg
Secretary Donna Shalala
Ms. Judith Feder
Assistant Secretary Philip Lee
Mr. Michel Lincoln
Arizona Congressional Delegation

THE INTER TRIBAL COUNCIL OF ARIZONA, INC.

Discussion Paper
THE IMPACTS OF INDIAN HEALTH SERVICE STAFFING AND BUDGET REDUCTIONS ON HEALTH SERVICES FOR INDIAN TRIBES
February 10, 1994

I. INTRODUCTION

The Clinton Administration has ordered the Indian Health Service (IHS) to reduce its staffing levels by 1,099 FTEs by the end of FY 1995. The staffing reductions will have a serious negative impact upon the ability of the IHS and tribal governments to provide health services on Indian lands.

President Clinton's proposed Health Security Act contains provisions which recognize the role of the Indian Health Service and tribal governments in the new national health care system. However, the IHS budget cuts proposed by the Clinton Administration will guarantee that the IHS and tribal governments will be unable to participate effectively in the national health care system.

II. RECOMMENDATIONS TO THE FEDERAL GOVERNMENT

A. Investing in Indian Health Care: A Four-Year Strategy

Instead of cutting the Indian Health Service budget, the Clinton Administration should adopt a plan to increase the annual IHS budget by 15 percent per year over a period of four years (fiscal years 1995-1999). The goal should be to fund the IHS at a level that will meet 100 percent of need as defined by the Indian Health Care Improvement Act.

The current IHS budget funds only 75 percent of Indian health care needs nationwide. A four-year strategy to invest in Indian health care would provide the IHS and tribal governments with the necessary resources to participate in the national health care system, as proposed in President Clinton's Health Security Act, when it is implemented in 1999.

B. Waivers for IHS FTE Reductions

The Office of Management and Budget should issue a waiver to the Indian Health Service from having to implement FTE reductions pursuant to Executive Order 12839. The Executive Order allows:

> ...exemptions necessary for the delivery of essential services and compliance with applicable law.

The Department of Health and Human Services has already applied for a waiver for IHS, but the waiver was denied by OMB. The Director of the Office of Management and Budget should approve the waiver.

C. Coordination of Clinton Administration Policy on Indian Health Care

The Clinton Administration's approach to Indian health care is uncoordinated. On one hand, the Administration includes IHS and tribal governments in its proposed Health Security Act. On the other hand, the Administration's budget would undermine the ability of the IHS and tribal governments to participate in the national health care system.

President Clinton should appoint a full-time staff person in the White House Office of Intergovernmental Affairs to coordinate the Clinton Administration's approach to Indian health care including IHS and tribal participation in health care reform, and the annual budget of the IHS.

D. Statutory Protections Against IHS Personnel Reductions

The Congress should restore appropriations language that was contained for many years in the Interior Appropriations Act protecting the Indian Health Service from FTE reductions:

> Provided further, That personnel ceilings may not be imposed on the Indian Health Service nor may any action be taken to reduce the full-time equivalent level of the Indian Health Service by the elimination of temporary employees by reduction in force, hiring freeze or any other means without the review and approval of the Committees on Appropriations.

E. The FY 1995 IHS budget

The Congress should reject the budget and FTE reductions proposed in the proposed FY 1995 IHS budget, as it did in the FY 1994 budget proposed by the Clinton Administration. The Congress should encourage the Clinton Administration to adopt the Four-Year Strategy to Invest in Indian Health Care.

III. BACKGROUND ON THE IHS FTE REDUCTIONS

A. Executive Order

President Clinton issued Executive Order 12839 on February 10, 1993, which called for a reduction of 100,000 Federal staff positions by the end of FY 1995. Each Federal agency was directed to reduce its personnel positions by 4 percent by the end of FY 1995.

On March 4, 1993, the Director of the Office of Management and Budget (OMB), Mr. Leon Panetta, issued OMB Bulletin 93-08 which contained instructions for Federal agencies to implement the FTE (full-time equivalent) reductions.

B. DHHS FTE Reductions Being Inequitably Imposed on the IHS

The Department of Health and Human Services (DHHS) had a total of 130,000 FTEs in FY 1993. The DHHS was ordered to reduce its total staffing by 5,200 FTEs by the end of FY 1995, a reduction of 4 percent.

The IHS had 15,426 FTEs in FY 1993. This represented 12 percent of all DHHS FTEs. The IHS was ordered to reduce its total staffing by 1,099 FTEs by the end of FY 1995, a reduction of 7 percent.

Compared against total DHHS FTE reductions (4 percent) the reduction of IHS FTEs (7 percent) is inequitable. The IHS is being directed to absorb one-fifth of the entire DHHS FTE reductions (1,099/5,200=21%).

The Assistant Secretary for Health, Dr. Philip Lee, required in his memorandum to the field that the FTE reductions to IHS were to be designed to minimize impact on patient care. Dr. Lee's December 8, 1993 memorandum on the hiring freeze specifically exempted staffing associated with essential patient care responsibilities. The result, in the Phoenix Area, is that the proposed reductions have been concentrated on housekeeping and dietary functions. However, health professionals cannot deliver quality health care in IHS hospitals that lack housekeeping and dietary services.

C. Contracting IHS Functions

The Public Health Service has justified a larger FTE reduction for IHS than the rest of the agency on the grounds that "the contracting/self-governance mechanism offered the opportunity to maintain services without adding Federal FTEs." One problem with the rationale is that the FTE reductions will be implemented long before tribal governments have an opportunity to conduct the planning necessary to contract for the functions that will be affected by the FTE reductions. Between the time that the FTE reductions are implemented and the Self-Determination contracts become effective, there would be a loss of services.

Tribal governments are not encouraged to enter into Self-Determination contracts in response to reductions in the Federal budget. Instead, budget cuts have the effect of discouraging tribal governments from contracting because Federal budget cuts send a message of a lack of Federal commitment for Indian health care.

The Clinton Administration should not try to impose major policy changes on Indian tribes in an environment of budget and FTE reductions. The first, and most sensible, reaction of Indian tribes is to protect the minimal level of resources that the

Federal government has provided for Indian health care.

IV. IMPACTS OF THE IHS FTE REDUCTIONS

A. The IHS is Inherently Labor Intensive

The IHS, either directly, or through Self-Determination contracts with tribal governments, provides health care on Indian lands nationwide through 50 hospitals, 158 health centers, 7 school clinics, 115 smaller health clinics and 173 Alaska village clinics.

The Phoenix Area Indian Health Service includes 41 tribal governments with lands located in Arizona, Nevada and Utah. There are 10 Service Units in the Phoenix Area. The IHS operates 7 inpatient hospitals in the Phoenix Area. In addition, the IHS operates the Phoenix Indian Medical Center (PIMC) which is a 147-bed regional referral center. The IHS also operates, either directly or through Self-Determination contracts with tribal governments, 15 health clinics and health stations.

The essential staff in IHS facilities includes doctors, dentists, pharmacists, nurses, laboratory staff, medical records staff, dietary staff and housekeeping staff. Health care is labor-intensive in general; it is more labor-intensive for rural Indian health care facilities which lack sophisticated and expensive diagnostic and treatment equipment.

B. The FTE reductions in the Phoenix Area

The Phoenix Area Indian Health Service has been ordered to reduce its staffing levels by 110 FTEs <u>by the end of FY 1994</u> and by another 64 FTEs by the end of FY 1995. In FY 1993, the total Phoenix Area staffing was 2,134 FTEs. The total reduction of 174 FTEs would result in a reduction of 8 percent of the Phoenix Area positions. On top of this, the Phoenix Area has been ordered to reduce another 23 FTEs because of an "administrative reduction."

There is no way that the IHS can implement a reduction of 197 FTEs in the Phoenix Area without crippling the ability of the IHS hospitals and clinics to function. The plan that has been developed by the IHS Phoenix Area Office would reduce 67 housekeeping positions and 72 dietary positions in 8 IHS hospitals. Although the plan proposes that the functions be contracted, the contracting of housekeeping and dietary functions in rural Indian communities is unrealistic.

C. The FTE Reductions will Further Diminish an Underfunded System

The Indian Health Care Improvement Act (PL 94-437, as amended) established a system of measuring the health care needs of Indian people and comparing the needs to the level of resources available to meet the needs. According to the methodology established pursuant to the Act, the IHS is funded at a level sufficient to meet approximately 75 percent of the health care needs of Indian reservation residents. On a national basis, the IHS programs were funded at the following levels in FY 1993:

Program	Level of Need Funded
Hospitals & Clinics	75 percent
Dental Services	44
Mental Health	54
Alcohol & Substance Abuse	44
Contract Health Care	75
Environmental Health	53
Public Health Nursing	33
Health Education	53
Community Health Reps.	43

The IHS FTE reductions will make the situation worse.

The Phoenix Indian Medical Center (PIMC) has been funded at less than 60 percent of need. The Congress provided additional funds in the FY 1994 Interior Appropriations Act to bring the PIMC up to 60 percent of need. The proposed cut of 63 FTEs from the PIMC housekeeping and dietary departments will result in a real loss of resources for the PIMC and the hoped-for progress in raising the level of health care resources will be lost.

V. HEALTH CARE REFORM AND THE IHS

A. President Clinton's Proposed Health Security Act

President Clinton's proposed Health Security Act is the only national health care reform proposal that addresses Indian health care and the role of the IHS and tribal governments. President Clinton's working group on health care reform is to be commended for recognizing the importance of the IHS and tribal health care system in the formulation of national health care policies.

Dr. Philip Lee, Assistant Secretary for Health, is conducting a series of regional meetings with tribal governments to discuss the Health Security Act with tribal governments. Dr. Lee is to be commended for taking the time to meet with tribal leaders and to learn more about tribal governments, the Indian Health Service and the concerns of tribal leaders.

B. Budget and FTE Reductions for IHS

However, the budget and FTE reductions that were proposed by the Clinton Administration in the FY 1994 IHS budget and that will be proposed in the FY 1995 IHS budget will undermine the ability of the IHS and tribal governments to function under the Health Security Act. In order to provide health care services to Indian reservation populations under the Health Security Act, the IHS and tribal governments will need to have in place health care delivery systems including health care personnel and facilities in rural communities. The proposed FTE reductions will virtually guarantee that the IHS will be unable to adequately serve Indian tribes.

If the IHS budget and FTEs continue to be cut during the next several years, the IHS and tribal governments will not able to provide the comprehensive benefits package under the Health Security Act. Given the geography, demographics and economics of Indian reservations, it is unlikely that other providers will be able to provide the comprehensive benefits package on Indian lands.

C. Lack of Coordination in the Clinton Administration

On one hand, the Clinton Administration is taking positive steps to work with tribal governments to strengthen the Indian health provisions in the Health Security Act. On the other hand, the Administration is proposing reductions in the IHS budget and staffing that would prevent the tribes and the IHS from effectively participating in the new health care system.

It appears that the "policy" side of the Clinton Administration is not coordinating with the "budget" side of the Administration with respect to Indian health care. The Clinton Administration should appoint an official in the White House Office of Intergovernmental Affairs to be responsible for coordinating the Administration's approach to Indian health care.

The Inter Tribal Council of Arizona, Inc.
February 10, 1994

Impact of Accross-the-Board FTE Reductions for — The Phoenix Area Indian Health Service

This is a response statement for percentage, across-the-board, FTE reductions as requested by IHS Headquarters.

Utilizing the fact the very earliest RIF/RIS could be implemented would be July 1, 1994 there is no way possible of meeting the requirements for FY 94. Therefore this will relate to the institution of reductions by the beginning of FY 95 so that the entire year will be included in the response to the FTE reductions.

I. The basic response, that will least affect the ability of the Service Units/Area Office to continue to meet their responsibilities, will be to contract for services currently being provided by federal employees. We have investigated this at several of our service units in the past and have found it NOT to be cost effective. However, it will reduce the federal payroll at the expense of providing less control and flexibility in meeting the needs of the facilities in the various locations. Also, as will be pointed out, it is doubtful if some of the services have vendors that could/would provide the necessary services to maintain the functions of the facility.

II. Required reductions and staffing are included in the following chart:

FTE Reduction Plan
Phoenix Area Indian Health Service

	FY '93 FTE	5.3% FY 94 Reduc	FTE Goal FY 94	4.1% FY 95 Reduc	FTE Goal - FY 95	Total Reductions
Area Office	256	14	242	10.	232	24
Colorado River	103	5	98	4	94	9
Ft. Yuma	79	4	76	3	73	7
Keams Canyon	132	7	125	5	120	12
Owyhee	82	4	78	3	74	8
PIMC	682	36	646	26	619	63
Sacaton	169	9	160	7	153	16
San Carlos	135	7	128	5	123	12
Schurz	70	4	66	3	64	6
U & O	51	3	48	2	46	5
Whiteriver	254	13	241	10.	231	23
NIH /1	54	3	51	2	49	5
Hqtrs /2	17	1	16	1	15	2
San Const. /3	32	2	30	2	29	3
Total	2,117	112	2,005	82	1,923	194

\1. Included in the Phoenix printouts and calculations are this number of positions for the NIH programs at PIMC and Sacaton.
\2. Included in the Phoenix printouts and calculations are this number of positions for Headquarters at CSC and Radiology.
\3. Included in this column are the positions currently in facilities construction. This figure varies depending on the number of and type of construction being done by the OEHE function throughout the Phoenix Area.

**** The figure to relate to on this chart is the totals in the line item "GOAL 95" (and/or "GOAL 94"). These lines relate to the same figures as given in the headquarters document for the respective periods. The beginning figures for "FTE 93" are calculated from the final automated report we received for fiscal year 93.

As mentioned above, we believe that the least disruptive method for dealing with the proposed reductions are to contract for the services required to carry on the direct care program at the Service Units. Contracting for most clinical professionals has proven to be neither affordable nor acceptable from a quality of care perspective. Therefore, we would suggest attempting the following as proposed guidelines for this process. (Obviously with this reduction there would remain the absolute requirement for RIF/RIS authority.) Impact statements, by activity, follow the chart.

FTE Reduction by Contracted Functions

		Required Reduction	Hskping	Dietary	Security	Transport.	CHS/ Bus Off.	Pharm	OHP	OPEIR
1.	Area Office	24			2				19	3
2.	Colorado River	9		4		2	3			
3.	Ft. Yuma	7	2	5						
4.	Keams Canyon	12	3	5	2	2				
5.	Owyhee	8	2	3		3				
6.	PIMC	63	31	32						
7.	Sacaton	16	8	8						
8.	San Carlos	12	6	6						
9.	Schurz	6					1	5		
10.	U & O	5	1				4			
11.	Whiteriver	23	14	9						
12.	NIH	5								
13.	Hqtrs	2								
14.	San Const.	3								
	Total	194	67	72	4	7	8	5	19	3

Notes:

1. Area Office: The plan would be to relocate the Office of Health Programs as a Division of the Office of Medical Center Services. This would be total conversion with each individual providing 1/3 time to direct care functions and 2/3 time to "Area" functions. The three positions in Program Planning that would be contracted are for the facilities planning and PJD/POR duties. This could possibly be contracted on an individual, site specific, basis. Undoubtedly this would create some problems with uniformity in products but this might be off-set by the individual attention given to each project. The security function of the Area Office could be contracted under the "buy Indian" regulations.

2. PIMC Service Unit: The two functions that could be contracted here are housekeeping and dietary. The major drawback to any contracting for dietary is that our employees have worked for years with traditional foods and education of the patients, so many of whom have type two diabetes and must use diet modification in order to control the onset of complications and the general deterioration that can occur with poor diabetic control. (**This will be referred to in all the proposals for dietary contracting.)

3. Keams Canyon Service Unit: Dietary - see #2.

4. Owyhee Service Unit: Dietary - see #2. In addition there is no identifiable contractor for these services. Therefore, we have indicated that the CHS/Business Office function might be more appropriate to consider for contracting. The problem with this is that very few outside entities are willing to deal with our "medical priorities" and other regulations.

5. Colorado River Service Unit: Dietary - see #2. CHS/Business Office - see #4.

6. Sacaton Service Unit: Dietary - see #2.

7. San Carlos Service Unit: Dietary - see #2.

8. Schurz Service Unit: There is a significant problem in this service unit as there is only one operation (Ft. McDermitt) that is IHS operated. The rest are (predominately) "638" contracts with employees under IPA or MOA assignment to the tribes. It is for that reason that we believe the least harmful contractible function may be pharmacy. There is one IHS employee whose main function is patient transport and this function could be contracted.

9. Whiteriver Service Unit: Dietary - see #2.

10. Ft. Yuma Service Unit: Dietary - see #2.

11. U & O Service Unit: CHS/Business Office - see #4.

12. National Institutes of Health: We do not feel authorized to indicate their proposal. However, we have been unable to receive their input because this information contained in the handouts is "embargoed" and not to be distributed.

13. Headquarters: This relates to the Clinical Support Center and the IHS Radiology function located here in Phoenix and counted in our printouts. We will not comment on their reductions except to say that an equal share should be borne by these operations.

14. Facilities Construction: We have no idea of the needs that may arise for emergency construction and what might be available through contracting.

These changes may be accepted by the local beneficiary and governmental constituencies but the overall impact on the direct care delivery of acute care services will be negatively impacted.

○

78-786 (320)